Mind Maps
for Medical
Students
Clinical Specialties

Mind Maps for Medical Students

Clinical Specialties

Olivia Smith
BSc (Hons), MSc (Dist)

The Hull York Medical School
Hull and York, UK

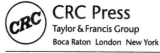

CRC Press
Taylor & Francis Group
Boca Raton London New York

CRC Press is an imprint of the
Taylor & Francis Group, an **informa** business

CRC Press
Taylor & Francis Group
6000 Broken Sound Parkway NW, Suite 300
Boca Raton, FL 33487-2742

© 2017 by Taylor & Francis Group, LLC
CRC Press is an imprint of Taylor & Francis Group, an Informa business

No claim to original U.S. Government works

Printed on acid-free paper

International Standard Book Number-13: 978-1-4987-8219-7 (Paperback)

Visit the Taylor & Francis Web site at
http://www.taylorandfrancis.com

and the CRC Press Web site at
http://www.crcpress.com

Contents

Please note due to the layout of the maps and tables, some pages within chapters have been left intentionally blank

For my father and mother.
This book is dedicated to my parents who have been the greatest influence in my life.
For all your unceasing encouragement, love and support I am forever grateful.

Medical students and trainees are faced with a huge volume of facts and knowledge that they must learn, assimilate and understand how to apply. Many hours are spent pouring over text books, online resources, lecture notes and papers. This tsunami of information is often hard to make sense of and the essentials difficult to remember.

Mind maps have become a popular way to help people understand complex interconnected concepts and information. Diagrams are used to visually organise information and show relationships among pieces of the whole. Despite technological advances, when it comes to efficient learning, simple methods, such as that used by Olivia Smith in *Mind Maps for Medical Students: Clinical Specialities*, can be highly effective.

Mind maps can take a lot of time to create. In this compact volume Olivia Smith, a senior medical student, has helped to do this for readers across eight core clinical specialities essential to the study of medicine. This is a sequel to her successful first book, *Mind Maps for Medical Students*, which distills a wide range of knowledge according to body systems. Both books organize a large amount of material in a logical, concise and conceptually appealing way to aid learning. By doing so it complements, but does not replace, more exhaustive sources and will also allow readers to position and contextualize new evidence as it emerges, so adding to their knowledge base.

It can be used by medical students, junior doctors and other health care professionals as a brief overview to introduce an area, for intense periods of revision and as an aide-mémoire. I hope this will encourage learners to develop their own mind maps in these or other areas and inspire other medical students to write.

Professor Trevor A Sheldon DSc, FMedSci
Dean, Hull York Medical School, UK

This book serves as a companion to *Mind Maps for Medical Students*. It aims to cover succinctly the main topics in clinical specialties that students and junior doctors are expected to be familiar with. It is a distillation of knowledge that aims to complement larger texts rather than replace them by presenting key facts in a digestible format. Each topic is presented in a logical manner following a design that may be utilized in OSCE assessments covering definitions, causes and investigations as well as treatments and complications. This will aid readers with their revision and consolidation of knowledge prior to examinations.

Wishing you all the very best in your examinations and future careers.

Olivia Smith BSc (Hons), MSc (Dist)
Final year medical student, The Hull York Medical School, UK.

ACE	angiotensin converting enzyme	**CRP**	C-reactive protein
ACE-III	Addenbrooke's Cognitive Examination	**CT**	computed tomography
		CTG	cardiotocography
ACL	anterior cruciate ligament	**DDH**	developmental dysplasia of the hip
ADHD	attention deficit hyperactivity disorder	**DIC**	disseminated intravascular coagulation
ADLs	activities of daily living	**DKA**	diabetic ketoacidosis
AIDS	acquired immunodeficiency syndrome	**DLQI**	Dermatology Life Quality Index
ALL	acute lymphoblastic leukaemia	**DM**	diabetes mellitus
ALT	alanine aminotransferase	**DMARD**	disease modifying antirheumatic drug
ANCA	antineutrophil cytoplasmic antibody	**DSM-5**	Diagnostic and Statistical Manual of Mental Disorders, 5th Edition
AP	anteroposterior		
APP	amyloid precursor protein	**DVT**	deep venous thrombosis
ARPKD	autosomal recessive polycystic kidney disease	**ECG**	electrocardiogram/ electrocardiography
ASD	atrial septal defect	**ECHO**	echocardiogram
ASO	antistreptolysin O	**ECT**	electroconvulsive therapy
AST	aspartate aminotransferase	**EEG**	electroencephalogram
BBPV	benign paroxysmal positional vertigo	**ELISA**	enzyme linked immunosorbent assay
BMI	body mass index	**EPSE**	extrapyramidal side effects
BP	blood pressure	**ESR**	erythrocyte sedimentation rate
BUN	blood urea nitrogen		
CADASIL	cerebral autosomal dominant arteriopathy with subcortical infarcts and leukoencephalopathy	**FBC**	full blood count
		FEV$_1$/FVC	forced expiratory volume in 1 second/fixed vital capacity
CBT	cognitive behavioural therapy	**FGFR3**	fibroblast growth factor receptor 3
CF	cystic fibrosis		
CFTR	cystic fibrosis transmembrane conductance regulator	**FIGO**	Fédération Internationale de Gynécologie et d'Obstétrique
CJD	Creutzfeldt–Jakob disease	**FSH**	follicle-stimulating hormone
CMV	cytomegalovirus	**GABA**	gamma-aminobutyric acid
COCP	combined oral contraceptive pill	**GAD-7**	Generalized Anxiety Disorder (Assessment)
COPD	chronic obstructive pulmonary disease	**GFR**	glomerular filtration rate
		GGT	gamma glutamyltransferase

GI	gastrointestinal	LDH	lactase dehydrogenase
GnRH	gonadotropin releasing hormone	LFTs	liver function tests
		LH	leutinizing hormone
HAART	highly active anti-retroviral therapy	LP	lumbar puncture
		MAO-B	monoamine oxidase type B (inhibitor)
HADS	Hospital Anxiety and Depression Scale	MAOI	monoamine oxidase inhibitor
hCG	human chorionic gonadotropin	MCV	mean corpuscular volume
HELLP	haemolysis, elevated liver enzymes, low platelet count (syndrome)	MMR	measles, mumps, rubella
		MND	motor neurone disease
		MRI	magnetic resonance imaging
HHV	human herpesvirus	NAAT	nucleic acid amplification test
HIV	human immunodeficiency virus	NEC	necrotizing enterocolitis
HPA	hypothalamic–pituitary–adrenal (axis)	NICE	National Institute for Health and Care Excellence
HPV	human papillomavirus	NICU	Neonatal Intensive Care Unit
HRT	hormone replacement therapy	NMS	neuroleptic malignant syndrome
HSP	Henoch–Schönlein purpura		
HSV	herpes simplex virus	NNRTI	non-nucleoside reverse transcriptase inhibitors
5-HT	5-hydroxytryptamine (receptors)	NRI	noradrenaline reuptake inhibitor
HUS	haemolytic uraemic syndrome	NSAID	non-steroidal anti-inflammatory drug
IBD	inflammatory bowel disease		
ICD-10	International Statistical Classification of Diseases and Related Health Problems, 10th Revision	NTD	neural tube defect
		OA	osteoarthritis
		OCD	obsessive compulsive disorder
IL	interleukin	PAS	pulmonary artery stenosis
IM	intramuscular	PASI	Psoriasis Area and Severity Index
IOP	intraocular pressure		
IUD	intrauterine device	PCL	posterior cruciate ligament
IUGR	intrauterine growth restriction	PCOS	polycystic ovary syndrome
		PCR	polymerase chain reaction
IUS	intrauterine system	PDA	patent ductus arteriosus
IV	intravenous	PEFR	peak expiratory flow rate
IVF	in-vitro fertilization	PET	positron emission tomography
LABA	long-acting beta agonist	PHQ-9	Patient Health Questionnaire
LCHAD	long-chain 3-hydroxyl-coenzyme A dehydrogenase	PID	pelvic inflammatory disease
		POP	progesterone only pill

PPH	post-partum haemorrhage	**SUFE**	slipped upper femoral epiphysis
PTSD	post-traumatic stress disorder	**TB**	tuberculosis
PUVA	psoralen + ultraviolet (A spectrum) light	**TCA**	tricyclic antidepressant
		TEN	toxic epidermal necrolysis
RA	rheumatoid arthritis	**TNM**	tumour/nodes/metastases (staging system)
RAST	radioallergosorbent test		
RBC	red blood cell	**TFTs**	thyroid function tests
RIMA	reversible inhibitor of monoamine oxidase A	**TOP**	termination of pregnancy
		TSH	thyroid stimulating hormone
RMI	Risk of Malignancy Index	**U&E**	urine and electrolytes
RUQ	right upper quadrant	**uE3**	oestriol
SABA	short-acting beta agonist	**UMN**	upper motor neuron
SFH	symphysis–fundal height	**USS**	ultrasound scan
SHBG	sex hormone binding globulin	**UTI**	urinary tract infection
SJS	Stevens–Johnson syndrome	**VDRL**	Venereal Disease Research Laboratory (test)
SNRI	serotonin noradrenaline re-uptake inhibitor	**VEGF**	vascular endothelial growth factor
SPECT	single-photon emission computed tomography		
		VMA/	(urinary) vanillyl mandellic
SSRI	selective serotonin re-uptake inhibitor	**pHVA**	acid/plasma homovanillic acid
		VSD	ventricular septal defect
STI	sexually transmitted infection	**VZV**	varicella zoster virus
SUDEP	sudden unexplained death in epilepsy	**WCC**	white cell count
		WHO	World Health Organization

Chapter One Psychiatry

Map 1.1. Depression

What is depression?

This is a condition of pervasive low mood. It is diagnosed using the ICD-10 or the DSM-5 and the following criteria need to be fulfilled:

1. Symptoms must be present for at least 2 weeks with a change from normal mood and at least two to three core symptoms.
2. Change in mood must not be secondary to drug or alcohol misuse, a medical condition or an adverse life event such as bereavement.
3. There must be impairment of social functioning.

Investigations

Ensure that the patient is really suffering from depression and not an organic disorder. This involves taking a careful history from the patient and the use of questionnaires such as HADS, PHQ-9, GAD-7 followed by investigations depending on patient presentation.

Always assess suicide risk.

- Baseline bloods: FBC, U&E, LFTs (including GGT and MCV for alcohol misuse), TFTs (hypothyroidism may cause low mood), ESR, glucose, calcium, vitamin B12 and folate levels.
- Specific tests are only used if indicated by history and examination (e.g. urine for toxicology, dexamethasone suppression test, syphilis serology etc).
- Radiology: CT or MRI may be indicated in some cases.

Causes

The cause is a complicated interaction between genetics, neurohormonal and psychosocial factors. A few examples are given below:

- Genetic: family history of depression.
- Neurohormonal: the monoamine hypothesis of depression is popular, which suggests that there are low levels of serotonin, noradrenaline and dopamine in the brain. Other theories include the suggestion of increased cortisol levels.
- Psychosocial: adverse life events and negative childhood experiences such as abuse, the loss of a parent and bullying. Chronic physical illness, unemployment and the lack of a confiding relationship are linked to increased rates of depression.

Treatment

Depends on the classification of depression. It includes psychological therapies such as CBT, antidepressants and ECT (see Table 1.1, p. 4)

MAP 1.1. Depression

Symptoms

These may be split into three broad categories: core symptoms, negative thinking and somatic symptoms:

Core symptoms: depressed mood, anergia, anhedonia.

Negative thinking: thoughts of guilt, low self esteem, thoughts of suicide and death, poor concentration.

Somatic symptoms: decreased weight (increased weight seen in atypical depression), sleep disturbance with early morning waking, decreased libido, constipation, psychomotor retardation or agitation.

These symptoms may be used to classify depression as mild, moderate or severe:

Classification	Presentation	Somatic or psychotic symptoms
Mild (4–5 symptoms)	Can continue with daily tasks	+/– somatic symptoms
Moderate (6–7 symptoms)	Real difficulty in completing daily tasks	+/– somatic symptoms
Severe (8–10 symptoms)	Unable to complete daily tasks	+/– psychotic symptoms

Psychotic symptoms are mood congruent or incongruent:

Mood congruent:
- Delusions: of poverty, guilt, punishment; if the patient holds the delusion that they are dead, then this is known as Cotard's syndrome.
- Hallucinations:
  - Auditory: usually derogatory voices.
  - Olfactory: rotting fruit/flesh.
  - Visual: tormentors.

Mood incongruent: thought insertion or withdrawal.

Map 1.1. Depression

Table 1.1. Treatment of depression

TABLE 1.1. **Treatment of depression. Treatment depends on the classification of depression.**

Classification of depression	Method of treatment
Mild	**Conservative therapy** This is a 'watchful waiting' approach and involves: An exercise regime: the current recommendations are three times a week for 45 minutes lasting 10–12 weeks • Alcohol and lifestyle advice • Sleep hygiene • Guided self help
Moderate – severe	**Conservative therapy:** • An exercise regime as above • Psychological therapies (e.g. cognitive behavioural therapy [CBT], which challenges the patient's thoughts and feelings in order to change them), counselling, interpersonal psychotherapy, dynamic therapy **Medical therapy:** • Antidepressants (see Table 1.2, p. 6). Most patients are started on an SSRI first line • If this initial therapy does not work, patients may be switched to alternative antidepressants, have their therapy augmented with antipsychotic or antiepileptic medication by a specialist or be referred for ECT (usually 6–12 sessions, twice weekly). The pathway followed depends on NICE and local guidance

Table 1.2. Antidepressants

TABLE 1.2. **Antidepressants.**

Class of antidepressant	Examples	Uses	Side effects
Selective serotonin reuptake inhibitors (SSRIs)	Citalopram Sertraline (often used in those who have previously had a myocardial infarction) Fluoxetine (has a long half-life) Paroxetine	DOBS: Depression OCD Bulimia Social phobias	• GI upset • Sexual dysfunction • Hyponatraemia in the elderly • Discontinuity syndrome: shivering, anxiety, headache, nausea, dizziness • Serotonin syndrome: muscle rigidity, seizures, cardiovascular collapse, hyperthermia. Treat serotonin syndrome with cyproheptadine (a 5-HT$_{2A}$ receptor antagonist)

Tricyclic antidepressants (TCAs)	Amitriptyline
	Imipramine
	Clomipramine
		DOBS:
		Depression
		OCD (clomipramine)
		Bed wetting (imipramine)
		Sometimes neuropathic pain (amitriptyline)
			• Linked to receptor blockade:
			  ○ α$_1$ antagonist: postural hypotension
			  ○ Antimuscarinic: dry mouth, urinary retention, constipation, blurred vision
			  ○ Antihistaminergic: weight gain, drowsiness
			• Toxicity = the **3Cs:**
			  Convulsions
			  Coma
			  Cardiotoxicity

Serotonin noradrenaline reuptake inhibitors (SNRIs)	Venlafaxine Duloxetine	Depression Generalized anxiety disorder (venlafaxine) Peripheral neuropathy (duloxetine)	• Increased blood pressure • Nausea • Sedation

Monoamine oxidase inhibitors (MAOIs)	Selegiline Moclobemide (reversible inhibitor of monoamine oxidase A [RIMA])	HAD: Hypochondriasis Anxiety Depression Selegiline is a MAO-B inhibitor that is licensed for use in Parkinson's disease	• Antimuscarinic: dry mouth, urinary retention, constipation, blurred vision • The Cheese Reaction – hypertensive crisis that occurs with ingestion of tyramine containing substances (e.g. cheese, pickled herring, soybean products, etc.)
α_2 antagonist	Mirtazapine	Depression PTSD	• Increased appetite and weight • Dry mouth • Sedation
Noradrenaline reuptake inhibitors (NRIs)	Reboxetine	DAP: Depression ADHD Panic disorder	• Antimuscarinic: dry mouth, urinary retention, constipation, blurred vision • Antihistaminergic: weight gain, drowsiness
Tetracyclics	Maprotiline	Depression	• Sedation • Postural hypotension

Table 1.2. Antidepressants

Map 1.2. Anxiety

What is anxiety?

Anxiety is a normal emotion that likely has been experienced by most of us during our lives. However, when anxiety is such that it interferes with daily functioning and performance, it is considered to be pathological. This relationship is called Yerkes–Dodson law.

Anxiety may be classified into many different subgroups:

Organic causes:
- Hyperthyroidism.
- Hypoglycaemia.
- Phaeochromocytoma.
- Cerebral trauma.
- Temporal lobe epilepsy.

Psychiatric causes:
- Anxiety disorders:
  - Phobic disorders (e.g. agoraphobia).
  - Non-situational disorders (e.g. generalized anxiety disorder [a triad of apprehension, motor tension and autonomic overactivity]).
  - Reaction to stressful events (e.g. PTSD).
  - OCD (see Map 1.3, p. 10).
- Secondary to depression or psychosis.
- Secondary to a medical condition.
- Secondary to psychoactive substance abuse (e.g. alcohol intake or withdrawal, amphetamines, benzodiazepine withdrawal).

Symptoms

These may be generalized or paroxysmal.

Remember as **PANICS**:
- **P** – Palpitations, pins & needles
- **A** – Abdominal discomfort
- **N** – Nausea and vomiting
- **I** – Intense fear of dying (angor animus)
- **C** – Chest pain, choking
- **S** – Sweating, swallowing difficulty (globus hystericus), shortness of breath

These symptoms may occur at different times and of varying intensity depending on the underlying disorder (e.g. if a patient had a social phobia, then an excessive anxious response would only occur on a specific social situation such as delivering a speech).

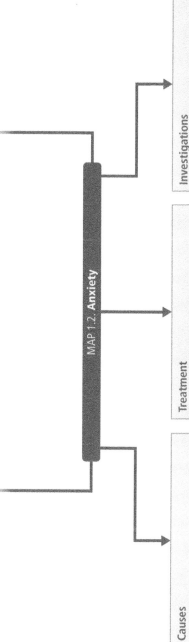

MAP 1.2. Anxiety

Causes

The genetic/biological model:
- Inherited disorder – many patients have a first-degree family relative with the disorder.
- Abnormal receptors in the 5-HT, noradrenaline and GABA systems.

The social/psychological model:
- Response to stressful life events.
- A psychologically susceptible patient may misinterpret a normal body stimulus.

Treatment

Depends on the type of anxiety disorder diagnosed, but consists of psychological and pharmacological therapy.

Psychological therapy:
- CBT.
- Behavioural therapy such as graded exposure.
- Psychodynamic therapy.

Pharmacological therapy:
- Antidepressants (see Table 1.2, p. 6).
- Anxiolytics (see Table 1.3, p. 12).

Investigations

There is no specific investigation for anxiety disorders, but it is vital to exclude an organic cause. Therefore, perform initial investigations:
- Bloods – FBC, U&E, TFTs, glucose, calcium levels.
- ECG.
- Toxicology report if indicated.
- Urinary VMA/pHVA if indicated (for phaeochromocytoma).

Map 1.2. Anxiety

Map 1.3   Obsessive compulsive disorder (OCD)

What is OCD?

OCD is a psychiatric disorder characterized by obsessive thoughts, ruminations and compulsive rituals. It affects men and women equally. The mean age of onset is 20 years.

The condition is associated with anankastic personality disorder, Gilles de la Tourette syndrome, depression and, less commonly, schizophrenia and basal ganglia disorders.

Treatment

Psychological therapy:

- CBT.
- Response prevention.
- Thought stopping.
- Cognitive modelling.

Pharmacological therapy:

- Antidepressants (see Table 1.2, p. 6), particularly clomipramine, which has strong anti-obsessional actions
- Anxiolytics (see Table 1.3, p. 12).
- Buspirone is used if marked anxiety present.

Psychosurgical:

- This is rare and only considered for intractable cases. Examples include stereotactic cingulotomy or yttrium radioactive implants.

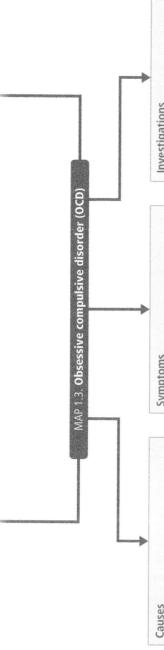

MAP 1.3. Obsessive compulsive disorder (OCD)

Causes

- Genetic factors: 3–7% of sufferers have a first-degree relative with the condition.
- Dysregulation/hypersensitivity of 5-HT receptors.
- Hyperactive orbitofrontal lobe.
- Basal ganglia dysfunction:
  ○ Dysfunctional striatum.
  ○ Smaller caudate nucleus.

Symptoms

Obsessive thoughts, compulsions, impulses, ruminations and rituals.

The ICD-10 highlights six features that are highly suggestive of the disorder:

1. Obsessions and compulsions that have been present for at least 2 weeks.
2. The obsessions and compulsions decrease the patient's function.
3. The patient is aware that these thoughts are generated from their own mind.
4. These thoughts are unpleasantly repetitive.
5. At least one of these thoughts is not resisted.
6. The compulsions and rituals performed are not, in themselves, pleasurable for the patient.

Investigations

There is no specific test for OCD. (See Map 1.2, p. 8, for tests required to rule out organic causes of anxiety and other types of anxiety disorder.)

Table 1.3. Anxiolytics and hypnotics

TABLE 1.3. Anxiolytics and hypnotics.

Drug name	Mechanism of action	Uses	Side effects
Buspirone	5-HT$_{1A}$ partial agonist	Generalized anxiety disorder	• Nausea and vomiting • Dizziness • Headache • Blurred vision
Amobarbital	Increases the inhibitory action of GABA by binding to the barbiturate binding site on the GABA$_A$ receptor. Increased influx of Cl$^-$ ions	Severe insomnia	• Dependence • Withdrawal symptoms • Daytime sedation • Cardiorespiratory depression • Drug interactions since it induces p450 system
Zolpidem	Binds to the benzodiazepine binding site on the GABA$_A$ receptor	Insomnia	• Dependence • Tolerance • Sedation • Drowsiness • Dizziness
Diazepam	Increases the inhibitory action of GABA by binding to the benzodiazepine binding site on the GABA$_A$ receptor. Increased influx of Cl$^-$ ions	Anxiety Insomnia Status epilepticus	• Dependence • Tolerance • Cardiorespiratory depression • Drowsiness • Sedation
Flumazenil	Competes at the benzodiazepine binding site. It is therefore an antagonist to the actions of zolpidem and diazepam	Benzodiazepine overdose	• Palpitations • Insomnia • Convulsion • Anxiety

Map 1.4. Schizophrenia

What is schizophrenia?

This is a chronic psychiatric disorder in which the patient experiences distorted reality. It affects men and women equally, although the former tend to have an earlier onset. The condition is associated with a higher suicide rate than the general population (10–15%).

Causes

The exact cause of schizophrenia is unknown but there are many theories:

1. The dopamine hypothesis – dopaminergic over activity.
2. Serotonergic overactivity – due to the superiority of clozapine in treating treatment resistant schizophrenia.
3. Genetics – higher incidence in those with a family history. Association with the *DISC1* gene (Disrupted In SChizophrenia).
4. Drug abuse – particularly cannabis use at an early age.
5. Group A personality disorder.
6. Illness during pregnancy.
7. Winter births.
8. Adverse life events.

Symptoms

The ICD-10 suggests that symptoms need to be present for at least 1 month.

These symptoms may be described as Schneider's first rank symptoms (remember as **TAP2**) or, more broadly, as positive and negative symptoms.

Schneider's first rank symptoms:

- **T** – Thought disorder – thought insertion, withdrawal, broadcasting. This may interfere with speech, leading to neologisms, thought stopping and knight's move thinking.
- **A** – Auditory hallucinations – thought echo, running commentary.
- **P** – Passivity phenomenon – belief that body is controlled by an external agency.
- **P** – delusional Perceptions – thinking an everyday object has a specific meaning for the patient.

Positive symptoms:

- Thought disorder – thought insertion, withdrawal, broadcasting.
- Delusions.
- Ideas of reference.

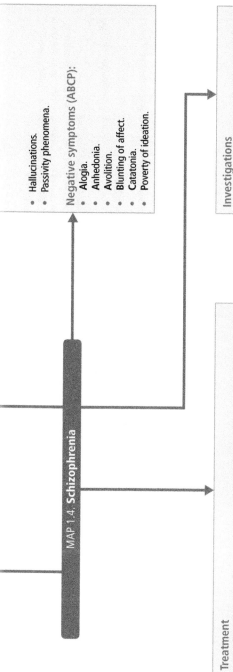

- Hallucinations.
- Passivity phenomena.

Negative symptoms (ABCP):
- Alogia.
- Anhedonia.
- Avolition.
- Blunting of affect.
- Catatonia.
- Poverty of ideation.

MAP 1.4. **Schizophrenia**

Investigations

There is no specific investigation for schizophrenia. It is a clinical diagnosis but it is vital to rule out other causes of psychosis, such as drug-induced psychosis, and to perform a risk assessment. Moreover, baseline bloods should be performed as well as an ECG due to the possible side effects of antipsychotic medication.

Treatment

Depends on whether it is an urgent or non-urgent situation. Follow your local guidelines.

Psychological therapy:
- CBT.
- Family intervention – prognosis is worse in families with high expressed emotion.
- Art therapy.
- Liaise with social worker regarding housing difficulties and employment.

Pharmacological therapy:
- Antipsychotics (see Table 1.4, p. 16).

Table 1.4. Antipsychotics

TABLE 1.4. Antipsychotics.

Classification	Examples	Mechanism of action	Uses	Side effects

Typical	Haloperidol Chlorpromazine Thioridazine	Block D$_2$ receptors, thereby increasing concentration of cAMP$_1$	Schizophrenia Psychosis Mania Tourette's syndrome	Antipsychotic medications block several receptors, which results in an array of side effects:
				
				• D$_2$ receptors affect several pathways:
				  ○ Tuberoinfundibular pathway: galactorrhoea, amenorrhoea, hyperprolactinaemia
				  ○ Nigrostriatal pathway: extrapyramidal side effects (EPSE). Remember as **TRAP**:
				  T – Tardive dyskinesia
				  R – Restless lower limbs (akathesia)
				  A – Acute dystonia
				  P – Parkinsonisms
				  ○ Mesocortical pathway: increases negative symptoms (see Map 1.4, p. 14).
				  ○ Mesolimbic pathway: decreases positive symptoms (see Map 1.4, p. 14).
				• α$_1$ antagonist: postural hypotension
				• Antimuscarinic: dry mouth, urinary retention, constipation, blurred vision
				• Antihistaminergic: weight gain, drowsiness
				• Neuroleptic malignant syndrome (NMS) – this is a life-threatening reaction that may be caused by an adverse reaction to antipsychotic drugs. Symptoms of NMS include: fever, muscle rigidity, altered mental status and autonomic dysfunction

Atypical	Olanzapine Clozapine Quetiapine Risperidone Aripiprazole	Block D_2 receptors thereby increasing concentration of $cAMP_1$ receptors, but are also effective in blocking $5\text{-}HT_2$, α_1 and H_1 receptors	Schizophrenia Olanzapine may also be used for anxiety disorders, OCD, mania, depression and Tourette's syndrome	• Side effects are the same as those listed for typical agents; however, there are far fewer EPSE and anticholinergic side effects, which is why atypical agents are preferred to the older, typical medications.
				• Specific side effects:
				  ○ Clozapine (used in treatment resistant schizophrenia): agranulocytosis
				  ○ Olanzapine: weight gain

Mood stabilizer	Lithium	Unknown. Thought to act in a similar way to other single charged cations by interfering with membrane ion transport mechanisms	Bipolar disorder Mania	• Common: tremor, diarrhoea, increased appetite • Those that require blood test monitoring: nephrogenic diabetes insipidus, hypothyroidism • In overdose: convulsions, coma, death • Teratogenic: Ebstein's abnormality • Special points: narrow therapeutic index. Monitor serum lithium concentration

Table 1.4 Antipsychotics

Map 1.5. Bipolar disorder

Types of bipolar disorder

Types	Key features
Bipolar I	• At least one manic episode lasting >1 week. • Usually coupled with periods of depression, but some patients may only have manic episodes.
Bipolar II	• >1 episode of severe depression, but only coupled with hypomania.
Rapid cycling	• >4 mood swings within a year.
Cyclothymia	• Mood swings that are not as severe as those in bipolar disorder. Follows a cyclic pattern that may last for longer periods.

Causes
The cause is a complicated interaction between genetic, neurohormonal, neuroanatomical and psychosocial factors. A few examples are given below:

Genetic: family history bipolar disorder. Possible involvement of chromosomes 6q and 8q21.

Neurohormonal: the monoamine hypothesis.

Neuroanatomical: increased size of lateral ventricles, abnormal HPA axis.

Psychosocial: adverse life events and negative childhood experiences such as abuse, PTSD.

What is bipolar disorder?
Major depression alongside at least one manic (bipolar I) or one hypomanic (bipolar II) episode characterizes this disorder. Patients will eventually suffer from depressive symptoms. In some ways this disorder may be viewed as a cyclical interchanging between elevated and low mood where the patient is functionally normal between episodes.

Men and women are equally affected.

MAP 1.5. **Bipolar disorder**

Treatment

Depends on whether it is an urgent or non-urgent situation. Follow your local guidelines.

Psychological therapy:
- CBT.
- Family focused therapy.
- Liaise with social worker regarding housing difficulties and employment.

Pharmacological therapy:
- Antipsychotics and mood stabilizers (see Table 1.4, p. 16).
- Antiepileptic medications are also used either independently or in combination with lithium.

Symptoms

- Those of depression (see Map 1.1, p. 2).
- Those of mania: these symptoms must be present for at least 1 week. Remember as **DIG FAST:**
  - **D** – Distractibility
  - **I** – Irresponsible behaviour (e.g. hedonistic behaviour without considering the consequences such as borrowing or spending vast sums of money and having unprotected sexual intercourse)
  - **G** – Grandiosity with delusions of power/wealth
  - **F** – Flight of ideas
  - **A** – Activity increases
  - **S** – Sleep decreases
  - **T** – Talkativeness

Investigations

- There is no specific investigation for bipolar disorder. It is a clinical diagnosis but it is vital to rule out other causes of psychosis, such as drug-induced psychosis, as well as organic mood disorders and to perform a risk assessment. Moreover, baseline bloods should be performed as well as an ECG due to the possible affects of antipsychotic medication. (**Note:** QTc prolongation may occur with all antipsychotics.)
- Investigations as for depression (see Map 1.1, p. 2).

Map 1.5. Bipolar disorder

Table 1.5. Personality disorders

TABLE 1.5. **Personality disorders. These are pervasive difficulties in personality that impact upon a patient's social functioning in a detrimental way. They are incredibly difficult to treat and often require years of psychotherapy.**

Cluster	General characteristics	Specific subtypes
A	Odd eccentric behaviour Do not form meaningful relationships Psychosis is not present	1. **Paranoid:** Suspicious Defence mechanism: projection 2. **Schizoid:** Social withdrawal/likes social isolation 3. **Schizotypal:** Eccentric behaviour and beliefs 'Magical thinking'
B	The emotional cluster Associated with mood disorders Associated with substance abuse	1. **Antisocial:** Affects males more than females Criminal behaviour and disregard for other members of society 2. **Borderline:** Affects females more than males Associated with depression Associated with deliberate self harm Feelings of emptiness Unstable interpersonal relationships Black and white thinking Impulsive behaviour Defence mechanism: splitting 3. **Histrionic:** Attention seeking, very flirtatious female Sexually provocative

		4. Narcissistic: Affects males more than females Grandiose delusions Lack of empathy Loves admiration and loathes criticism
C	The anxious cluster Associated with anxiety disorders	**1. Avoidant:** Very sensitive to rejection Avoids social situations **2. Anankastic:** Associated with OCD Perfectionist personalities **3. Dependent:** Low self esteem 'Clingy'

Table 1.5 Personality disorders

Map 1.6. Anorexia nervosa

What is anorexia nervosa?

This is an eating disorder that is characterized by ICD-10 by four key points:

1. BMI <17.5.
2. Self-induced weight loss.
3. A morbid fear of fatness.
4. Endocrine dysfunction (e.g. amenorrhoea).

This condition affects females 10–20 times more than males. It is associated with social classes I and II as well as certain professions (e.g. models and dancers).

Causes

The cause is a complicated interaction between genetics, neurohormonal and psychosocial factors. A few examples are given below:

- Genetic: family history of anorexia nervosa.
- Neurohormonal: abnormalities in serotonin metabolism.
- Psychosocial: adverse life events, perfectionist personalities, high achieving families, media expectations of thinness relating to the ideal female form.

Treatment

Psychoeducation concerning weight and nutrition.

Psychological therapy:
- CBT.
- Family focused therapy.
- Interpersonal therapy.
- Psychodynamic therapy.

Pharmacological therapy:
- Correction of electrolyte imbalance.
- Restore healthy weight.
- Prescribe meals that are nutritionally appropriate.

Urgent situations may require refeeding under the Mental Health Act.

MAP 1.6. Anorexia nervosa

Symptoms

- Excessive weight loss.
- Weakness and fatigue.
- Cold peripheries.
- Bradycardia.
- Hypotension.
- Amenorrhoea.
- Thin lanugo hair over face and body.
- Inability to perform squat test.
- Co-morbid depression/OCD.

Signs

- Signs of induced purging:
  - Russell's sign.
  - Tooth enamel that is pitted/eroded.
  - Enlarged parotid glands.
- Signs of electrolyte imbalance:
  - Cardiac arrhythmias.

Complications

- Death.
- Endocrine dysfunction (e.g. amenorrhoea).
- Metabolic alkalosis – from excessive vomiting.
- Metabolic acidosis – from laxative abuse.
- Cardiac complications (e.g. arrhythmias and QT prolongation that may lead to sudden death).
- Refeeding syndrome – results in hypophosphataemia, which can lead to rhabdomyolysis, arrhythmias, respiratory failure, convulsions, coma and death.
- Electrolyte abnormalities – hypokalaemia, hyponatraemia, hypoglycaemia, hypocalcaemia, hypercholesterolaemia.
- Anaemia.
- Proximal myopathy.

Investigations

Clinical assessment: overall clinical assessment including the use of tools such as the **SCOFF** questionnaire:

S – Have you ever made yourself **S**ick because you are uncomfortably full?

C – Do you feel that you have lost **C**ontrol over how much you eat?

O – Have you lost **O**ne stone in a 3 month period?

F – Do you believe yourself to be **F**at when others say you are thin?

F – Does **F**ood dominate your life?

- BMI = weight (kg)/height (m)^2.
- Bloods – FBC, U&E, LFTs, TFTs, glucose, calcium levels.
- ECG.
- Blood pressure.
- Toxicology report if indicated.

Map 1.6 Anorexia nervosa

Map 1.7. Bulimia nervosa

What is bulimia nervosa?

This is an eating disorder that is characterized by ICD-10 by three key points:

1. Patient engages in binge eating.
2. There is evidence of purgative behaviour (e.g. vomiting to counteract the effects of binge eating and increased weight).
3. A morbid fear of fatness.

Causes

The cause of bulimia is unclear, but it is thought to be due to complex interactions between genetic, neurohormonal and psychosocial factors. A few examples are given below.

Genetic: family history of bulimia nervosa.

Neurohormonal: theories involving alteration of serotonin and noradrenaline exist.

Psychosocial: adverse life events, perfectionist personalities, past dieting behaviour, anorexia nervosa, personality disorders particularly borderline patients, low self esteem and depression.

Symptoms

- Remember that patients may actually be overweight due to binge eating behaviour.
- Co-morbid depression/OCD.

Signs

- Signs of induced purging:
  ○ Russell's sign.
  ○ Tooth enamel that is pitted/eroded.
  ○ Enlarged parotid glands.
  ○ Oesophageal tears.
- Signs of electrolyte imbalance:
  ○ Cardiac arrhythmias.
  ○ Hypokalaemia is associated with vomiting as well as laxative abuse.

MAP 1.7. Bulimia nervosa

Treatment

Psychological therapy:
- CBT.
- Family focused therapy.
- Interpersonal therapy.
- Psychodynamic therapy.

Pharmacological therapy:
- Correction of electrolyte imbalance.
- Antidepressants such as TCAs and SSRIs have been shown to decrease purgative behaviour.

Urgent situations are less common than for anorexia nervosa since patients are often of normal weight.

Investigations

Like anorexia nervosa, there is no specific underlying test for bulimia nervosa. However, it is important to rule out organic causes of weight gain and weight loss as well as performing a psychiatric evaluation. It is important to perform the investigations listed below, particularly U&E, since electrolyte disturbances are common with purgative behaviour.

- BMI = weight (kg)/height $(m)^2$.
- Bloods – FBC, U&E, LFTs, TFTs, glucose, calcium levels.
- ECG.
- Blood pressure.
- Toxicology report if indicated.

Map 1.8 Attention deficit hyperactive disorder (ADHD)

What is ADHD?

This is pervasive, developmentally inappropriate behaviour in which the patient lacks concentration and is hyperactive. It is more common in males than females and must be present in at least two different settings (e.g. at home and at school). The symptoms must be present for at least 6 months.

Causes

The cause is a complicated interaction between genetics, neurohormonal and psychosocial factors. A few examples are given below.

Genetics: possible involvement of chromosomes 5, 6 and 11.

Neurohormonal: dysregulation of dopamine and noradrenaline.

Psychosocial: familial dysfunction, parental stress, potentially food additives.

Complications

- Substance misuse.
- Dissocial personality disorder.
- Unemployment.
- Low self esteem.
- Increased rate of suicide.

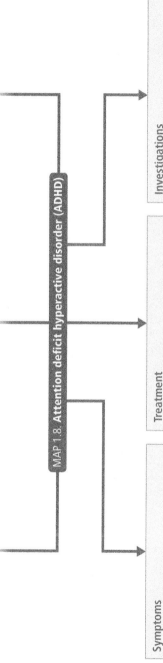

MAP 1.8. **Attention deficit hyperactive disorder (ADHD)**

Symptoms
- Decreased concentration.
- Poor school performance.
- Forgetfulness.
- Hyperactive behaviour.
- Inability to organize tasks.
- Fidgeting.
- Very talkative.
- Often interrupts.

Treatment
Psychological therapy:
- CBT.
- Family focused therapy including parent management therapy.
- Educational intervention.

Pharmacological therapy:
- Methylphenidate (Ritalin) is the treatment of choice.

Investigations
- There is no specific test for ADHD, but it is important to perform a full developmental, medical and familial assessment as well as obtaining information from the child's school concerning their behaviour.
- The Conners Comprehensive Assessment Scale may aid initial assessment and follow-up appointments.

Map 1.8 Attention deficit hyperactive disorder (ADHD)

TABLE 1.6. Dementia. Dementia is a syndrome of a progressive global decline in cognitive function.

Type of dementia	Causes	Signs and symptoms	Investigations	Treatment	Complications

Alzheimer's disease	Exact cause unknown. Risk factors include:
	• Down's syndrome due to ↑ amyloid precursor protein (APP) gene load
	• Familial gene associations:
	  ○ APP – chromosome 21
	  ○ Presenilin-1 – chromosome 14
	  ○ Presenilin-2 – chromosome 1
	  ○ Apolipoprotein E4 (APoE4) alleles – chromosome 19
	• Hypothyroidism
	• Previous head trauma
	• Family history of Alzheimer's disease
		• Amnesia
		• Disorientation
		• Changes in personality
		• Decreasing self care
		• Apraxia
		• Agnosia
		• Aphasia
		• Lexial anomia
		• Paranoid delusions
		• Depression
		• Wandering
		• Aggression
		• Sexual disinhibition
			Mental state examination and mini-mental state examination
			Addenbrooke's cognitive examination (ACE-III)
			FBC, U&E, LFTs, TFTs, CRP, ESR, glucose, calcium, magnesium, phosphate, VDRL, HIV serology, vitamin B_{12} and folate levels, blood culture, ECG, chest x-ray, CT, MRI, SPECT
			Three main findings on histology: **BAT**
			B – Beta amyloid plaques
			A – ↓ Acetylcholine
			T – neurofibrillary Tangles
				• Memantine – inhibits glutamate by blocking NMDA receptors
				• Donepezil – acetylcholinesterase inhibitor
				• Rivastigmine – acetylcholinesterase inhibitor
					• Amnesia
					• Increased risk of infection
					• Dysphagia
					• Urinary incontinence
					• Increased risk of falls

Table 1.6. Dementia

| Vascular dementia | • Is the second most common cause of dementia
• Caused by infarcts of small and medium sized vessels in the brain
• Genetic association with cerebral autosomal dominant arteriopathy with subcortical infarcts and leukoencephalopathy (CADASIL) on chromosome 19 | Follows a deteriorating stepwise progression. There are three types:
1. Vascular dementia following stroke
2. Multi-infarct dementia following multiple strokes
3. Binswanger disease following microvascular infarcts
• Amnesia
• Disorientation
• Changes in personality
• Decreasing self care
• Depression
• Signs of UMN lesions (e.g. brisk reflexes)
• Seizures | Mental state examination and mini-mental state examination
Addenbrooke's cognitive examination (ACE-III)
FBC, U&E, LFTs, TFTs, CRP, ESR, glucose, calcium, magnesium, phosphate, VDRL, HIV serology, vitamin B_{12} and folate levels, cholesterol levels, vasculitis screen, syphilis serology, ECG, chest x-ray, CT, MRI, SPECT | • Dietary advice
• Smoking cessation
• Treat DM and hypertension
• Aspirin | Significant co-morbidity (e.g. cardiovascular disease and renal disease) |

Continued overleaf

Table 1.6. Dementia

TABLE 1.6. Dementia. Dementia is a syndrome of a progressive global decline in cognitive function (continued).

Type of dementia	Causes	Signs and symptoms	Investigations	Treatment	Complications
Dementia with Lewy bodies	• Associated with Parkinson's disease • Avoid antipsychotic drugs in these patients	Is a triad of: 1. Parkinsonism – bradykinesia, gait disorder 2. Hallucinations – predominately visual, usually of animals and people 3. Disease process follows a fluctuating course	Mental state examination and mini-mental state examination Addenbrooke's cognitive examination (ACE-III) CT, MRI, SPECT ApoE genotype Lewy bodies, ubiquitin proteins and alpha-synuclein found on histology	• AVOID ANTIPSYCHOTICS – cause hypersensitivity to neuroleptics • Levodopa may be used to treat Parkinson's symptoms but these may worsen psychotic symptoms	• Neuroleptic hypersensitivity • Autonomic dysfunction • Fluctuating blood pressure • Arrhythmias • Urinary incontinence • Dysphagia • Increased risk of falls
Frontotemporal dementia (Pick's disease)	• Genetic association with chromosome 17q21–22 and tau gene 3 mutations	• Amnesia • Disorientation • Changes in personality • Decreasing self care • Mutism • Echolalia • Overeating • Parkinsonism • Disinhibition	Mental state examination and mini-mental state examination Addenbrooke's cognitive examination (ACE-III) CT, MRI, SPECT	Currently none. Only supportive treatment available.	• Increased risk of falls • Increased risk of infection

Table 1.6 Dementia

		Histology: depends on subtype: 1. Microvacuolar type – microvacuolation 2. Pick type – widespread gliosis, no microvacuolation 3. MND type – histological changes like MND	
Huntington's dementia	• Caused by Huntington's disease, which is an autosomal dominant disorder where there is a defective gene on chromosome 4 • Causes uncontrollable choreiform movements and dementia	Uncontrollable choreiform movements	Diagnostic genetic testing	No cure. Treat symptoms: • Chorea – an atypical antipsychotic agent • Obsessive compulsive thoughts and irritability – SSRIs	• Dysphagia • Increased risk of falls • Increased risk of infection

Continued overleaf

Table 1.6. Dementia

TABLE 1.6. **Dementia. Dementia is a syndrome of a progressive global decline in cognitive function** (continued).

Type of dementia	Causes	Signs and symptoms	Investigations	Treatment	Complications
Creutzfeldt–Jakob disease (CJD)	• Caused by prions • Progressive and without cure • There is also variant CJD (vCJD), which has an earlier onset of death	• Rapidly progressive dementia (4–5 months) • Amnesia • Disorientation • Changes in personality • Depression • Psychosis • Ataxia • Seizures	EEG – triphasic spikes seen LP – for 14-3-3 protein CT, MRI	No cure	• Increased risk of infection • Coma • Heart failure • Respiratory failure
Other causes	• HIV • Vitamin B_{12} deficiency • Syphilis • Wilson's disease – autosomal recessive condition where copper accumulates within the tissues • Dementia pugilistica (aka "punch drunk" syndrome) – seen in boxers and patients who suffer multiple concussions				

Table 1.6. Dementia

Table 2.1: UK antenatal booking appointments

TABLE 2.1: **UK antenatal booking appointments. Useful website that summarizes the current programme: http://cpd. screening.nhs.uk/flashvideo/NHSPregnancyScreening.mp4.**

Gestation	What happens during the appointment?
8–12 weeks	This is the initial booking appointment: • Take a general history enquiring about past medical maternal history and maternal lifestyle factors including alcohol, smoking and diet. Also, ask about folic acid and vitamin D supplementation. Start these supplements if they are not being taken • Measure blood pressure • Perform a urine dip stick and culture (for asymptomatic bacteriuria) • Measure patient's BMI • Routine blood tests: FBC, blood group, rhesus status, red blood cell alloantibodies • Screen for infectious disease: HIV, hepatitis B, rubella, syphilis
10–13 + 6 weeks	• Date confirming scan • Screens for multiple pregnancy
11–13 + 6 weeks	• Down's syndrome screening: the combined test is offered to women 11–14 weeks gestation. This consists of the nuchal translucency scan and blood tests (serum beta human chorionic gonadotropin and serum pregnancy-associated plasma protein A)
16 weeks	• Routine blood test: FBC – give iron supplementation if anaemic • Measure blood pressure • Perform a urine dip stick and culture
18–20 + 6 weeks	• Fetal anomaly scan
25 weeks	Only for primiparous mothers: • Measure symphysis–fundal height (SFH) • Measure blood pressure • Perform a urine dip stick and culture

28 weeks	• Measure SFH • Measure blood pressure • Perform a urine dip stick and culture • Routine blood test: FBC – give iron supplementation if anaemic. Check for atypical red blood cell alloantibodies • Give anti-D prophylaxis to rhesus-negative mothers
31 weeks	Only for primiparous mothers: • Measure SFH • Measure blood pressure • Perform a urine dip stick and culture
34 weeks	• Measure SFH • Measure blood pressure • Perform a urine dip stick and culture • Give anti-D prophylaxis to rhesus-negative mothers • Counsel mother about birthing plan and specific wishes or concerns
36 weeks	• Measure SFH • Measure blood pressure • Perform a urine dip stick and culture • External cephalic version for breech presentations • Counsel mother about breast feeding and post-natal depression/baby blues
38 weeks	• Measure SFH • Measure blood pressure • Perform a urine dip stick and culture

Continued overleaf

Table 2.1: UK antenatal booking appointments

TABLE 2.1. UK antenatal booking appointments. Useful website that summarizes the current programme: **http://cpd.screening.nhs.uk/flashvideo/NHSPregnancyScreening.mp4** (*continued*).

Gestation	What happens during the appointment?		
40 weeks	• Measure SFH • Measure blood pressure • Perform a urine dip stick and culture • Counsel mother about induction of labour		
41 weeks	• Measure SFH • Measure blood pressure • Perform a urine dip stick and culture • Counsel mother about induction of labour		

TABLE 2.2. **The physiology of labour. There are three stages of labour and the success of each stage depends on maternal, fetal and mechanical factors.**

Stage of labour	Subcategories	Approximate duration	Specific investigations
1. Onset of contractions until full dilatation of the cervix	1. Latent stage – until the cervix reaches 4 cm 2. Active stage – from 4–10 cm	Variable	Measure fetal heart rate using CTG Measure maternal heart rate, blood pressure and temperature
2. From full dilatation of the cervix until the delivery of the fetus	May be split into a passive and an active stage. The fetus mechanically follows a pathway to be expelled from the uterus. This pathway is as follows: 1. The head becomes engaged 2. The fetus descends to 'station zero' (the level of the ischial spines) 3. Head flexion 4. Head rotates internally 5. Head extends 6. Head rotates externally 7. Shoulders and body are subsequently delivered	2–3 hours	Measure fetal heart rate using CTG Measure maternal heart rate, blood pressure and temperature
3. From delivery of the fetus until delivery of the placenta	Note umbilical cord lengthening	30 minutes	Measure fetal response using the APGAR score Check maternal vital signs

Table 2.2. The physiology of labour

Table 2.3: Dystocia

TABLE 2.3. Dystocia. In layman's terms this means difficult childbirth. There are many reasons why childbirth may be difficult and these may be classified into maternal causes, fetal causes and mechanical causes. Some examples are presented below.

Maternal factors	Fetal factors	Mechanical factors
Ineffective uterine contraction: this often occurs in nulliparous women who have had a prolonged labour **Maternal illness** (e.g. diabetes mellitus, pre-eclampsia, eclampsia) **Problematic placental implantation** (e.g. placenta praevia)	**Fetal malpresentation** **Macrosomia:** associated with maternal diabetes	**Cephalopelvic disproportion:** there are four broad anatomical types of female pelvis: • Gynecoid • Android • Anthropoid • Platypelloid **Shoulder dystocia:** this has a variety of associations such as diabetes mellitus, macrosomia, small maternal size and a past obstetric history of shoulder dystocia. To manage this problem several manoeuvres may be employed starting with the McRobert's manoeuvre. Others include the Wood's screw procedure and the Zavanelli manoeuvre

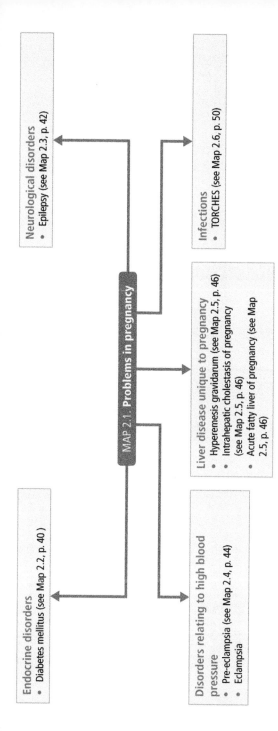

MAP 2.1. **Problems in pregnancy**

Endocrine disorders
- Diabetes mellitus (see Map 2.2, p. 40)

Neurological disorders
- Epilepsy (see Map 2.3, p. 42)

Disorders relating to high blood pressure
- Pre-eclampsia (see Map 2.4, p. 44)
- Eclampsia

Liver disease unique to pregnancy
- Hyperemesis gravidarum (see Map 2.5, p. 46)
- Intrahepatic cholestasis of pregnancy (see Map 2.5, p. 46)
- Acute fatty liver of pregnancy (see Map 2.5, p. 46)

Infections
- TORCHES (see Map 2.6, p. 50)

Map 2.1. Problems in pregnancy

Map 2.2. Diabetes mellitus (DM) in pregnancy

What is diabetes mellitus in pregnancy?

This is metabolic condition in which the patient has hyperglycaemia due to insulin insensitivity or decreased insulin secretion.

Causes

These may be:

Pre-existing. There are many – only a few common causes are listed here:

- Type 1 DM: this is an autoimmune condition, which results in the destruction of the pancreatic beta cells resulting in no insulin production. This condition has a juvenile onset and is associated with HLA-DR3 and HLA-DR4. Patients are at risk of ketoacidosis.

- Type 2 DM: this occurs when patients gradually become insulin resistant or when the pancreatic beta cells fail to secrete enough insulin, or both. It usually has a later life onset; however, the incidence is increasing in young populations due to environmental factors such as increasing obesity and sedentary lifestyle. Patients are at risk of developing a hyperosmolar state.

- Chronic pancreatitis: this condition destroys both alpha and beta pancreatic cells so that glucagon and insulin are no longer produced and secreted.

Symptoms

- General: polyuria, polyphagia, polydipsia, blurred vision, glycosuria, signs of macrovascular and microvascular disease.
- More common in type 1 DM: acetone breath, weight loss, Kussmaul breathing, nausea and vomiting.

MAP 2.2.
Diabetes mellitus (DM) in pregnancy

Investigations

Diagnostic investigations for DM are:

- Fasting plasma glucose: >7 mmol/L (126 mg/dL).
- Random plasma glucose (plus DM symptoms): >11.1 mmol/L (200 mg/dL).
- HbA1C: >6.5%.

Other tests include:

- Impaired glucose tolerance test (for borderline cases):
  ○ Fasting plasma glucose: <7 mmol/L (126 mg/dL) and at 2 hours a level of 7.8–11 mmol/L (140–200 mg/dL)
  ○ Plasma glucose at 2 hours: >11.1 mmol/L (>200 mg/dL)
- Impaired fasting glucose:
  ○ Plasma glucose: 5.6–6.9 mmol/L (110–126 mg/dL).

Specific to gestational DM:

- Oral glucose tolerance test at 16–18 weeks and at 28 weeks if initial test is normal.
- Gestational diabetes may be diagnosed when the blood glucose level is >9 mmol/L 2 hours after a 75 g oral glucose load.

Complications

General:
- Macrovascular: hypertension, increased risk of stroke, myocardial infarction, diabetic foot.
- Microvascular: nephropathy, neuropathy (glove and stocking distribution), retinopathy.
- Psychological: depression.

Fetal:
- Neural tube and cardiac defects.
- Macrosomia and shoulder dystocia.
- Neonatal hypoglycaemia.

Maternal:
- DM later in life.
- Potentially instrumental delivery or caesarean section.

Gestational (i.e. it developed during pregnancy). This often normalizes after the baby is delivered but many women go on to develop DM later in life. The exact cause of gestational diabetes is unknown. It is associated with many risk factors such as high maternal BMI, ethnic origin with a high prevalence in those with South Asian ancestry, a previous history of gestational diabetes or a macrosomic baby (weight >4.5 kg).

Treatment (gestational DM specific)

Conservative:
- Ensure that mother is under consultant led care.
- Ensure mother is taking a higher dose of folic acid (5 mg/day) due to an increased risk of neural tube defects.
- Diet control.
- Increased exercise.

Medical:
- Metformin.
- Insulin.

Map 2.2. Diabetes mellitus (DM) in pregnancy

What is epilepsy?

This is a condition in which the brain is affected by recurrent seizures.

Causes

Seizures are caused by abnormal paroxysmal neuronal discharges in the brain, which are usually a result of some form of traumatic brain injury. These discharges display hypersynchronization. The causes of epilepsy may be broadly classified into three types:

1. Idiopathic – cause for epilepsy is unknown.
2. Cryptogenic – cause for epilepsy is unknown, but there are signs that suggest that the cause may be linked to brain injury (e.g. patient has autism or learning difficulties).
3. Symptomatic – cause known. Some causes of symptomatic epilepsy include: **VINDICATE:**

V – Vascular: history of stroke
I – Infection: history of meningitis or malaria
N – Neoplasms: brain tumour
D – Drugs: alcohol and illicit drug use
I – Iatrogenic: drug withdrawal
C – Congenital: family history of epilepsy
A – Autoimmune: vasculitis
T – Trauma: history of brain injury
E – Endocrine: ↓Na⁺, ↓Ca²⁺, ↓ or ↑ glucose

Investigations

Note that epilepsy will often be diagnosed before the lady falls pregnant. However, the following tests are used to help aid the diagnosis of epilepsy and identify the cause.

- Bloods – FBC, U&E, LFTs, CRP, ESR, glucose, calcium levels
- Radiology – MRI
- Other – ECG, LP, EEG

Signs and symptoms

These depend on the region of the brain affected.

- Frontal lobe: JAM:
  J – Jacksonian march.
  A – pAlsy (post-ictal Todd's palsy).
  M – Motor features.

- Temporal lobe: ADD FAT:
  A – Aura that the epileptic attack will occur.
  D – Déjà vu.
  D – Delusional behaviour.
  F – Fear/panic – *hippocampal involvement.*
  A – Automatisms.
  T – Taste/smell – *uncal involvement.*

- Parietal and occipital lobes:
  Visual and sensory disturbances

Others include: partial or generalized seizures with or without convulsions, tongue biting, migraines and depression.

MAP 2.3. Epilepsy in pregnancy

Treatment (pregnancy specific)

Continuing antiepileptic therapy during pregnancy is advisable since the risks of having seizures while pregnant outweigh the harm of therapy on the fetus.

Conservative:
- Ensure that mother is under consultant led care.
- Ensure mother is taking a higher dose of folic acid (5 mg/day) due to an increased risk of neural tube defects.

Medical:
- Neonatal care – vitamin K injection.
- Carbamazepine is considered to be the least teratogenic of the older antiepileptic agents.
- Sodium valproate has the strongest association with neural tube defects.

Complications (pregnancy specific)

General:
- Injuries while having seizure.
- Depression.
- Anxiety.
- Brain damage.
- Sudden unexplained death in epilepsy (SUDEP).

Fetal:
- Neural tube defects (associated with sodium valproate especially).
- Cleft palate (associated with phenytoin).
- Intrauterine growth restriction.
- Developmental delay.

Map 2.3. Epilepsy in pregnancy

Map 2.4. Pre-eclampsia

What is pre-eclampsia?

This is a multisystemic disorder characterized by four factors:

1. Hypertension >140/90 mmHg.
2. Occurs after 20 weeks gestation.
3. Proteinuria >0.3 g/24 hours.
4. Normalizes after delivery of fetus.

Causes

It is a placental disease but the exact pathogenesis is incompletely understood. Pre-eclampsia is, however, associated with numerous risk factors such as:

- Extremes in age: <20 or >40 years.
- Nulliparity.
- Multiple pregnancy.
- New partner.
- Past history of pre-eclampsia.
- High maternal BMI.
- Previous hypertension.
- Previous renal disease.
- Previous DM.
- Interval between pregnancies >10 years.

Symptoms

- May be asymptomatic.
- Headache.
- Visual disturbance.
- Abdominal pain (typically right upper quadrant or epigastric region).
- Nausea and vomiting.

Investigations

- Monitor fetal distress using CTG.
- Bloods – FBC, U&E, LFTs, glucose (particularly screening for HELLP syndrome), uric acid level.
- Measure blood pressure: >140/90 mmHg.
- Urinalysis: proteinuria.
- Neurology examination: hyperreflexia, clonus.
- Fundoscopy: papilloedema.

MAP 2.4. Pre-eclampsia

Complications

Fetal:
- Intrauterine growth restriction.
- Premature delivery.

Maternal:
- Eclampsia.
- HELLP syndrome.
- Cerebral haemorrhage.
- Intra-abdominal haemorrhage.

Treatment

Delivery is the definitive treatment of pre-eclampsia but other options are employed while the fetus develops. Follow NICE/consensus guidelines.

Conservative:
- Patient education.
- Regular blood pressure monitoring.

Medical:
- Labetalol is used first line.
- Other agents include nifedipine and hydralazine.
- Magnesium sulphate is also used for seizure prevention.

Map 2.4. Pre-eclampsia

Map 2.5. Liver disease unique to pregnancy

MAP 2.5. Liver disease unique to pregnancy

Hyperemesis gravidarum

What is hyperemesis gravidarum?
This is a complication of pregnancy, which begins during the first trimester and usually resolves by week 20. A triad characterizes the condition:

1. Nausea and vomiting.
2. Weight loss (5% or more of pre-pregnancy body weight).
3. Dehydration.

Causes
The exact cause is unknown.

Symptoms
- Nausea and vomiting.
- Weight loss (5% or more of pre-pregnancy body weight).
- Dehydration – resulting in ketosis and constipation.
- Metabolic imbalance – ketosis and thyrotoxicosis.
- Hyperolfaction.
- Ptyalism.

Investigations
- Monitor fetal distress using CTG.

Intrahepatic cholestasis of pregnancy

What is intra-hepatic cholestasis of pregnancy?
This is a reversible hormonally influenced cholestasis, which typically presents during the second trimester and continues into the third trimester.

Causes
The exact cause is unknown. Studies have suggested that this condition is linked to increased hormone levels. Increased risk with multiple pregnancies. This condition often recurs in subsequent pregnancies.

Symptoms
- Pruritus, typically commencing on the palms of the hands and soles of the feet. Itching then spreads to the face and trunk. Worse at night. No rash present.
- Jaundice.
- Steatorrhoea.

Investigations
- Monitor fetal distress using CTG.

- Bloods – FBC, U&E, BUN, TFTs (TSH low), LFTs = AST, ALT <1,000 IU/L, ALT>AST, vitamin B levels.
- Urinalysis.
- USS – monitor gestation and exclude molar pregnancy (see Map 3.3, p. 76).

Treatment

Medical:
- IV fluid resuscitation.
- Antiemetics – pyridoxine, promethazine.
- Nutritional support – thiamine.

Complications

Mother:
- Weight loss.
- Complications of vomiting (e.g. oesophageal rupture, renal damage, vascular depletion, Wernicke's encephalopathy).

Fetus:
- Prematurity.
- Low birth weight.

- Bloods – FBC, U&E, BUN, LFTs = AST, ALT <1,000 IU/L, GGT normal, bile acid levels (high), prothrombin (normal), bilirubin <6 mg/dL.
- Urinalysis.
- USS – monitor gestation.

Treatment

- Medical: ursodeoxycholic acid, antihistamines.
- Delivery of fetus (usually at 37 weeks or when fetal distress is imminent).

Complications

Mother:
- Severe pruritus – interferes with sleep.
- Deranged clotting – due to decreased vitamin K levels.

Fetus:
- Fetal distress.
- Stillbirth.
- Meconium ingestion/aspiration.

Map 2.5 Liver disease unique to pregnancy

Map 2.5. Liver disease unique to pregnancy

MAP 2.5. **Liver disease unique to pregnancy** (*continued*).

Acute fatty liver of pregnancy

What is acute fatty liver of pregnancy?

This is a serious complication of pregnancy that typically occurs in the third trimester. It is characterized by microvesicular steatosis (variant form of hepatic fat accumulation) in the liver. Associated with eclampsia.

Causes

The exact cause is unknown. Increased risk in women who have a heterozygous long-chain 3-hydroxyacylcoenzyme A dehydrogenase (LCHAD) deficiency. This condition is thought to be due to mitochondrial dysfunction. Dysfunction of the mitochondria results in the dysfunction of fatty acid oxidation and, as such, an accumulation of fat within the hepatocytes. Excess fat infiltration results in acute hepatic insufficiency.

Symptoms

- Non-specific – lethargy, nausea and vomiting.
- Hypertension.
- Abdominal pain – epigastric, RUQ.
- Symptoms associated with: upper gastrointestinal haemorrhage, acute kidney injury, pancreatitis, hypoglycaemia, fulminant hepatic failure.
- Encephalopathy – altered mental status and confusion.
- Jaundice.

Investigations

- Monitor fetal distress using CTG.

- Bloods – FBC, platelets <100,000 mm^3, fibrinogen level (low), antithrombin III, U&E, BUN, LFTs = AST, ALT >300 IU/L, prothrombin (increased), bilirubin (increased), DIC, glucose levels (decreased).
- Urinalysis.
- Maternal USS – liver (increased echogenicity).
- Fetal USS – monitor gestation.

Treatment

Medical:
- Resuscitation – IV fluids, IV glucose, fresh frozen plasma, cryoprecipitate.
- Delivery of fetus.

Surgical:
- Liver transplant may be required for mothers with severe liver failure, encephalopathy or severe DIC.

Complications

Mother:
- Fulminant hepatic failure.
- DIC.
- Encephalopathy.
- Death <20%.

Fetus:
- Fetal mortality ~45%.

Map 2.6. TORCHES infections

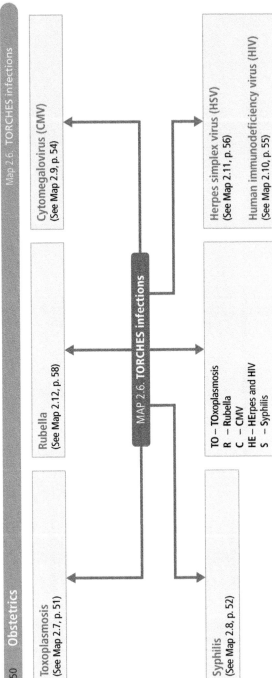

Toxoplasmosis
(See Map 2.7, p. 51)

Rubella
(See Map 2.12, p. 58)

Cytomegalovirus (CMV)
(See Map 2.9, p. 54)

MAP 2.6. **TORCHES infections**

Syphilis
(See Map 2.8, p. 52)

TO – **TO**xoplasmosis
R – **R**ubella
C – **C**MV
HE – **HE**rpes and HIV
S – **S**yphilis

Herpes simplex virus (HSV)
(See Map 2.11, p. 56)

Human immunodeficiency virus (HIV)
(See Map 2.10, p. 55)

What is toxoplasmosis?

This is an infection caused by *Toxoplasma gondii*, a protozoan. Infection is more common in immunosuppressed individuals (e.g. HIV, cancer sufferers).

Transmission:
- Infected meat.
- Cat faeces.

Symptoms
- Often asymptomatic.
- Flu-like symptoms – fatigue, sore throat, headache, fever, lymphadenopathy.

Complications

Fetal: Remember as the 3Cs:
- **C** – Cerebral manifestations (e.g. hydrocephalus, microcephaly).
- **C** – Convulsions.
- **C** – Chorioretinitis.

Maternal: Remember as **ABCDE**:
- **A** – Abscess formation (cerebral)
- **B** – Blurred vision
- **C** – Confusion
- **D** – Difficulty breathing (pneumonitis)
- **E** – Encephalomyelitis

MAP 2.7. **Toxoplasmosis**

Treatment

Conservative:
- Patient education.
- Advise pregnant women to avoid cats/clearing litter trays.
- Do not allow pet cat to sleep in same bed.
- Highlight hand hygiene, especially if handling raw meat.

Medical:
- Fetal:
  ○ Pyrimethamine.
  ○ Sulphonamide.
- Maternal:
  ○ Spiramycin.

Investigations
- Blood test: maternal immunoglobulin M.
- Radiology: ultrasound scan for fetal hydrocephalus.
- Amniocentesis.
- Perform additional tests (e.g. for HIV co-infection if clinically relevant).

Map 2.7. Toxoplasmosis

What is rubella?

This is a single stranded RNA virus. It is also known as German measles. Greatest risk of infection and complications is during the first few weeks of pregnancy.

Transmission:

- Airborne infection passed through respiratory droplets.

Symptoms

- Arthralgia.
- Sore throat.
- Fever.
- Macular rash – initially on face but spreads to torso and then legs. Duration about 3 days.
- Occipital lymphadenopathy; this may be painful and cause discomfort.

Investigations

- Blood test: maternal antibodies.
- Urinalysis: for virus in neonate.

MAP 2.8. **Rubella**

Treatment

There is no specific treatment for rubella.

Conservative:
- Patient education.
- Advise pregnant women to avoid known contacts with rubella (e.g. known cases at work).

Medical:
- Maternal:
  - MMR vaccine.

Complications

Fetal:
- Congenital rubella syndrome - remember as **ABCDE**:
  - **A** – A small head (microcephaly) and low birth weight
  - **B** – Blueberry muffin rash (extramedullary haematopoiesis)
  - **C** – Congenital heart malformations (PDA, PAS)
  - **D** – Deafness (sensorineural)
  - **E** – Eye abnormalities (cataracts)

Maternal: as in Symptoms box.

Map 2.8. Rubella

Map 2.9. Cytomegalovirus (CMV)

Symptoms
- Generally asymptomatic.

Investigations
- Blood test: maternal antibodies.
- Radiology: USS may show hyperechogenic bowel.
- Hyperechogenic bowel is also found in cystic fibrosis and Down's syndrome.

Complications
Fetal: remember as **ABCDE:**
A – A small head microcephaly) and low birth weight
B – Blindness (occasionally)
C – Causes neonatal jaundice
D – Deafness (high risk)
E – Enlarged liver and spleen

Maternal: as in Symptoms box.

MAP 2.9. **Cytomegalovirus (CMV)**

What is CMV?
This is an enveloped virus belonging to the Herpesviridae family.

Transmission:
- Airborne infection passed through respiratory droplets.
- Via maternal genitourinary tract.

Treatment
There is no specific treatment for CMV.
The medications used to treat CMV ordinarily are teratogenic.

Conservative:
- Patient education.

Medical:
- **Maternal:**
  - Consider termination of pregnancy.

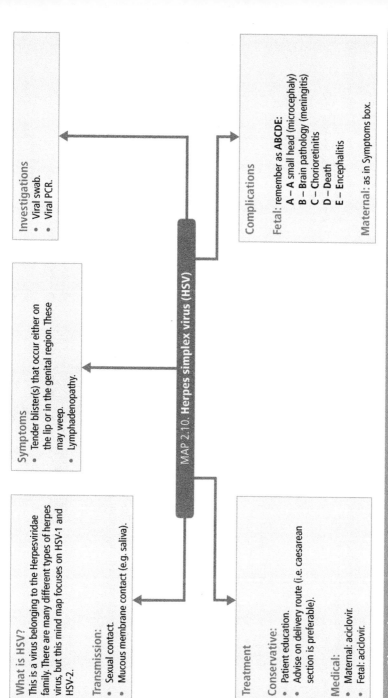

Investigations
- Viral swab.
- Viral PCR.

Complications

Fetal: remember as **ABCDE**:
  A – A small head (microcephaly)
  B – Brain pathology (meningitis)
  C – Chorioretinitis
  D – Death
  E – Encephalitis

Maternal: as in Symptoms box.

Symptoms
- Tender blister(s) that occur either on the lip or in the genital region. These may weep.
- Lymphadenopathy.

MAP 2.10. Herpes simplex virus (HSV)

What is HSV?
This is a virus belonging to the Herpesviridae family. There are many different types of herpes virus, but this mind map focuses on HSV-1 and HSV-2.

Transmission:
- Sexual contact.
- Mucous membrane contact (e.g. saliva).

Treatment

Conservative:
- Patient education.
- Advise on delivery route (i.e. caesarean section is preferable).

Medical:
- Maternal: aciclovir.
- Fetal: aciclovir.

Map 2.11. Human immunodeficiency virus (HIV)

What is HIV?
This is an RNA retrovirus of the Lentivirus genus. This virus causes acquired immunodeficiency syndrome (AIDS).

Cause
There are two types of HIV:
- HIV-1:
  - Group M, subtypes A to J: prevalent in Europe, North America, Australia and sub-Saharan Africa.
  - Group O: mainly in Cameroon.
- HIV-2:
  - Predominantly confined to West Africa.

Transmission
- Unprotected sexual intercourse.
- Shared needles (e.g. drug users).
- Contaminated blood tranfusions.
- Vertical transmission – mother to child. The virus crosses the placenta and is transmitted through breast milk.

Genes required for viral replication
PEG:

P – pol: encodes reverse transcriptase and integrase

E – env: encodes envelope proteins (e.g. gp120)

G – gag: encodes viral structural proteins.

Investigations
- Enzyme-linked immunosorbent assay (ELISA).
- Western blot test.
- Immunofluorescence assay (IFA).
- Nucleic acid testing.

MAP 2.11. **Human immunodeficiency virus (HIV)**

Treatment

Conservative:

- Patient advice, planned caesarean delivery, infant bottle feeding.

Medical:

- Highly active antiretroviral therapy (HAART):
  - Nucleoside reverse transcriptase inhibitors (NRTIs) (e.g. zidovudine [particularly to reduce vertical transmission]). **Note:** Zidovudine is the only agent shown to decrease perinatal transmission.
  - Non-nucleoside reverse transcriptase inhibitors (NNRTIs) (e.g. nevirapine).
  - Protease inhibitors (PIs) (e.g. atazanavir).
- Give either:
  - Two NRTIs combined with one NNRTI; or
  - Two NRTIs combined with one PI; or
  - Two NRTIs combined with one integrase inhibitor (II; e.g. raltegavir).

Special notes:

- NRTIs cross the placenta, the NNRTIs nevirapine and efavirenz cross the placenta, but PIs do not cross the placenta easily.
- Zidovudine is given intravenously during labour.
- Neonatal care: infant zidovudine, initiated as soon as possible after delivery and continued until 6 weeks.
- Hepatitis B co-infections: tenofovir and lamivudine or emtricitabine.

Complications

Fetal:

- IUGR.
- Stillbirth.

Maternal:

- Pre-eclampsia.
- Increased risk of infection:
  - Toxoplasmosis.
  - CMV retinitis.
  - *Pneumocystic jirovecii* pneumonia.
  - Kaposi's sarcoma.
  - Cryptococcal meningitis.
  - *Mycobacterium avium* complex.

Map 2.12. Syphilis

MAP 2.12. **Syphilis**

What is syphilis?
This is a sexually transmitted disease caused by the spirochaete *Treponema pallidum*.

Transmission:
- Sexual contact.

Symptoms
Infections occurs in three stages:
1. Chancre – painless.
2. Disseminated disease – rash on palms and soles.
3. Cardiac and neurological involvement.

Investigations
- Venereal Disease Research Laboratory (VDRL) test.
- Rapid plasma reagin test.
- Fluorescent treponemal antibody absorption test (FTA-ABS).
- *Treponema pallidum* haemagglutination test (TPHA).
- *Treponema pallidum* particle agglutination test (TPPA).
- Treponemal enzyme immunoassay (EIA).

Treatment

Conservative:
- Patient education.
- Advise on delivery route (i.e. caesarean section is preferable)

Medical: (many antibiotics listed below are contraindicated during pregnancy. Consult local guidelines and the BNF). Mother may need to consider termination of pregnancy.

- Maternal:
  - Procaine penicillin G.
  - Doxycycline.
  - Erythromycin.
  - Azithromycin.

Note: If patient has neurosyphilis, give prophylactic prednisolone to avoid the Jarisch–Herxheimer reaction. This reaction may occur after antibacterial treatment, which causes the death of the spirochaete and subsequent endotoxin release. Endotoxins cause the Jarisch–Herxheimer reaction.

- Fetal:
  - Penicillin.

Complications

Fetal: ABCDES:
- A – A small head (microcephaly)
- B – Brain pathology (meningitis). Blood stained nasal discharge
- C – Choroiditis
- D – Dental malformations, Deafness (sensorineural)
- E – Enlarged liver and spleen
- S – Skin lesions, Seizures

Maternal:
- Miscarriage.
- Gumma formation.
- Meningitis.
- Stroke.
- Heart valve damage.

Map 2.13. Placental abruption

What is placental abruption?

This is a cause of antepartum haemorrhage, which may be defined as vaginal bleeding that occurs at <24 weeks gestation. The causes of antepartum haemorrhage may be remembered as **PVC**[2]:

P – Placental abruption
P – Placenta praevia
V – Vasa praevia
V – Vaginal infection
C – Cancer of the cervix
C – Cervicitis

Causes

Placental abruption occurs when the placenta separates from the wall of the uterus. It is subclassified as either a concealed or revealed (more common) abruption.

Risk factors

Remember as **OH PIPS**:

O – Overdistended uterus
H – Hypertension

P – Pre-eclampsia
I – Intra-uterine growth restriction
P – Past history of placental abruption
S – Smoking history

Symptoms

- Vaginal bleeding.
- Severe abdominal pain out of keeping with blood loss, coupled with signs of systemic shock may indicate concealed abruption.
- Wooden uterus on palpation.

Investigations

- Monitor fetal distress with CTG.
- Blood tests: FBC, U&E, group and save.
- Radiology: USS for placenta praevia.

MAP 2.13. **Placental abruption**

Treatment

Medical:
- Emergency treatment: admission, cross-match and blood transfusion.
- Consider delivery depending on gestation. If the fetus is <34 weeks, giving steroids to the mother will help induce fetal lung development.

Complications

Fetal:
- Death
- Intra-uterine growth restriction

Maternal: DADS:
- **D** – Death
- **A** – Acute kidney injury
- **D** – Disseminated intravascular coagulation and multi-organ failure
- **S** – Shock

Map 2.13. Placental abruption

Map 2.14. Placenta praevia

Symptoms

- Painless vaginal bleeding.
- Abnormal fetal lie/failure of engagement.

Investigations

- Monitor fetal distress with CTG.
- Blood tests: FBC, U&E, group and save.
- Radiology: abdominal and transvaginal USS.

What is placenta praevia?

This is a 'low lying placenta' and a cause of antepartum haemorrhage, which may be defined as vaginal bleeding that occurs at <24 weeks gestation. Other causes of antepartum haemorrhage are listed in Map 2.13, p. 60.

Placenta praevia may be classified as either minor or major. The major form completely covers the internal os, whereas in the minor form the internal os is only partially covered.

Causes

Placenta praevia is caused by low implantation of the embryo.

Risk factors

Remember as **MUMS:**
M – Maternal age
U – Uterine abnormality
M – Multiparity
S – Section (caesarean)

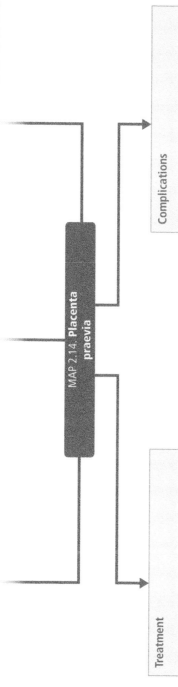

MAP 2.14. **Placenta praevia**

Complications

Fetal:
- Death
- Premature delivery.

Maternal:
- Massive haemorrhage and death.
- Hysterectomy.
- High risk of post-partum haemorrhage.

Treatment

Medical:
- Emergency treatment: admission, cross-match and blood transfusion.
- Consider elective caesarean section depending on gestation. If the fetus is <34 weeks, giving steroids to the mother will help induce fetal lung development.

What is PPH?

This is bleeding that occurs after delivery of the fetus. It may be defined as primary, secondary or massive depending on the amount of blood lost and the time that has elapsed post delivery.

Type of PPH	Blood lost	Time elapsed after birth
Primary	>500 mL	<24 hours
Secondary	>500 mL	>24 hours to 12 weeks
Massive	>1,500 mL	N/A

Causes

Primary: remember as the 5Ts:

    T – Tone of uterus lost (most common cause)

    T – Trauma (e.g. to perineum or uterine rupture)

    T – Torn cervix or vagina

    T – Thrombin (i.e. bleeding disorders)

    T – Tissue (i.e. retained products of conception)

Secondary:

- Infection – endometritis.
- Retained products of conception.

Risk factors: remember as ABCD:

    A – Antepartum haemorrhage

    B – Birthing problems (i.e. instrumental delivery, induced labour)

    C – Coagulation disorders (e.g. von Willebrand disease)

    D – Duration of labour >12 hours

Symptoms

Depends on the cause of PPH. All may present with shock:

- Atonic uterus: uterus is enlarged.
- Uterine rupture: abdominal pain, vaginal blood loss.
- Infection: tachycardia, fever, abdominal pain, vaginal blood loss.
- Retained conception products: signs of infection (see above).

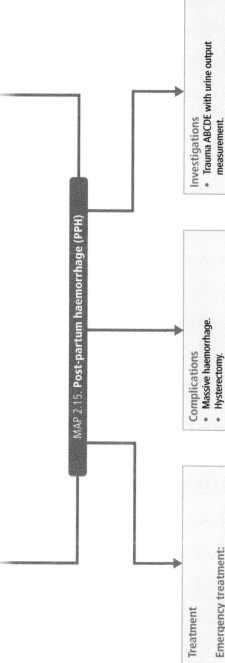

MAP 2.15. Post-partum haemorrhage (PPH)

Investigations
- Trauma ABCDE with urine output measurement.
- Identify cause (e.g. vaginal examination).
- Monitor fetal distress with CTG.
- Blood tests: FBC, U&E, group and save.
- Radiology: abdominal and transvaginal USS.

Complications
- Massive haemorrhage.
- Hysterectomy.
- Death.

Treatment
Emergency treatment:
- Generally resuscitation management including an ABCDE approach with insertion of two wide bore cannulas.
- Bloods: cross-match and blood transfusion.
- Specific management depending on cause:
  - Atonic uterus: uterine massage.
  - Uterine rupture: laparotomy.
  - Endometritis: antibiotics (check local guidelines).
  - Retained products of conception: evacuation with suction curette.

Map 2.15. Post-partum haemorrhage (PPH)

Map 2.16. Rhesus disease

What is rhesus disease?

This disease is one cause of haemolytic disease of the newborn. Antibodies from a rhesus-negative mother destroy fetal blood cells, resulting in haemolytic disease.

Causes

Rhesus disease occurs as a direct result of maternal antibodies attacking fetal blood cells. This happens when the mother is rhesus negative but the fetus is rhesus positive. The mother must have been previously sensitized (by exposure to rhesus-positive blood [e.g. during a previous pregnancy]).

Symptoms

Symptoms depend on the severity of rhesus disease.

Blood lost	Time elapsed after birth
Mild	Mild anaemia Moderate jaundice
Moderate	Moderate anaemia Moderate–severe jaundice
Severe	Severe anaemia Hydrops foetalis Hypoglycaemia

General symptoms:
- Hypotonia.
- Off feeds.
- Haemolytic anaemia (of varying severity).
- Jaundice (of varying severity).

Investigations

- Rhesus status is diagnosed during the routine UK screening programme (see Table 2.1, p. 34).
- Coombs test – blood sampling from the umbilical cord assesses baby's blood type as well as whether anti-D antibodies have passed into the baby's blood.

MAP 2.16. **Rhesus disease**

Complications

- Haemolytic disease of the newborn.
- Stillbirth.
- Learning difficulties.
- Deafness.
- Blindness.

Treatment

Medical:

- Preventing rhesus disease:
  - Routine antenatal anti-D prophylaxis:
    1. Single dose treatment – at 28–30 weeks.
    2. Double dose treatment – at 28 weeks and 34 weeks.
  - Anti-D immunoglobulin given at any sensitizing event (e.g. any bleeding).
  - Anti-D immunoglobulin given within 72 hours after birth if mother has not been sensitized.
- Treating rhesus disease:
  - Phototherapy.
  - Intravenous immunoglobulin.
  - Blood transfusions.

Map 2.16. Rhesus disease

Map 2.17. Symphysis pubis dysfunction

What is symphysis pubis dysfunction?

This is a condition of pain and discomfort that occurs in some pregnant women due to increased movement and misalignment of the pelvic bones at the pubis symphysis. Symptoms tend to worsen as the pregnancy progresses and there is an increased risk with multiparity.

Causes

Due to increased laxity of the pelvic ligaments. This occurs due to increased relaxin hormone levels.

Symptoms

- Pain and pelvic discomfort (typically at the pubic symphysis but may also occur at the sacroiliac joints).
- Pain worsens with movement and certain activities such as climbing stairs.
- Waddling gait.
- Palpation – tenderness over the pubic symphysis; a gap may be felt.

Investigations

- Usually a clinical diagnosis.
- Radiology – USS may be used to assess the degree of separation at the pubic symphysis. 9 mm is considered physiological in pregnancy; >10 mm in pregnancy is considered pathological.

MAP 2.17. Symphysis pubis dysfunction

Complications

- Diastasis of the symphysis pubis.

Treatment

Conservative:
- Physiotherapy.
- Place a pillow between the legs while in bed resting.
- Avoid activities that worsen the pain.

Medical:
- Analgesia: paracetamol.

TABLE 2.4. Breastfeeding.		
Advantages	**Disadvantages**	**Absolute contraindications**
Benefits for baby: • Decreased risk of infection (e.g. chest infection, ear infection, urinary tract infection) • Decreased risk of asthma • Decreased risk of eczema • Decreased risk of diabetes mellitus • Decreased risk of diarrhoea and vomiting **Benefits for mother:** • Decreased risk of cancer: breast and ovarian • Decreased risk of osteoporosis • Increased bonding with child	• Vertical transmission • Risk of mastitis • Mother requires additional calories	• Vertical infections (e.g. HIV) • Galactosaemia • Drugs: remember **ABCS**: A – Antibiotics (e.g. tetracyclines) A – Aspirin A – Amiodarone B – Benzodiazepine C – Cytotoxic drugs C – Carbimazole S – Sulphonylureas

Table 2.4. Breastfeeding

Map 3.1. Ectopic pregnancy

What is an ectopic pregnancy?

This is when the embryo implants outside the uterus. The embryo may implant in the abdomen but more often it is a tubal pregnancy most commonly located in the ampulla region of the fallopian tube (80%).

Causes

Anything that narrows or damages the fallopian tube may result in an ectopic pregnancy.

Remember as **TIPS**:

T – The progesterone only pill – results in thickened secretions.

I – Infection and IVF treatment.

P – Pelvic inflammatory disease.

S – Surgical procedures – result in adhesions.

Symptoms

Consider in any sexually active female who has abdominal pain and who has missed a period:

- Abdominal pain – usually in the lower right or lower left quadrants and colicky in nature.
- Vaginal bleeding – dark coloured and likened to 'prune juice'.
- Nausea and vomiting.
- Signs of shock: clammy appearance, pale, tachycardic, hypotensive.
- Vaginal examination: cervical excitation.

Investigations

- Pregnancy test and β-hCG levels.
- Blood tests: FBC, U&E, group and save.
- Radiology: transvaginal USS.

MAP 3.1. **Ectopic pregnancy**

Complications

Remember as **TUBE**:

T – Tubal rupture.

U – sUbfertility.

B – Blues (i.e. psychological implications related to child loss and possible subfertility).

E – Ectopic pregnancy risk increases for subsequent pregnancies.

Treatment

Emergency treatment

Depends on initial presentation:

- General resuscitation management including an ABCDE approach with insertion of two wide bore cannulas.
- Bloods: cross-match and blood transfusion.
- Consider anti-D prophylaxis.

Medical:

- Methotrexate.

Surgical:

- Laparoscopic salpingotomy/salpingectomy.
- If this fails, then consider laparotomy.

Map 3.2. Miscarriage

What is a miscarriage?

This is when the fetus is spontaneously aborted <24 weeks gestation, with the majority being <12 weeks gestation. There are many different types of miscarriage. These may be defined as either complete or incomplete, or classified according to their presentation, such as inevitable, threatened, missed and recurrent.

Causes

Mostly the cause is unknown but broad causes, particularly of recurrent miscarriage, may be remembered as **ABC**:

A – Antiphospholipid syndrome, increasing Age
B – Bleeding disorders (e.g. von Willebrand disease)
C – Chromosomal abnormality, Cervical incompetence

Symptoms

Symptoms depend on the type of miscarriage.

Type of miscarriage	Symptoms	Cervical os open or closed
Inevitable	Heavy vaginal bleeding Abdominal pain	Open
Threatened	Light vaginal bleeding Fetus may survive	Closed
Missed	No vaginal bleeding Fetus is no longer viable	Closed

Investigations

- β-hCG levels.
- Blood tests: FBC, U&E, group and save, rhesus status.
- Radiology: transvaginal USS.

MAP 3.2. Miscarriage

Complications

- Infection and pyrexia.
- Psychological implications including depression.
- Complication of surgical curettage (e.g. the risk associated with general anaesthetic, uterine perforation, Asherman's syndrome [intrauterine adhesions]).

Treatment

- Depends on clinical presentation and the type of miscarriage.

Emergency treatment:

- May be required if mother is haemorrhaging.

Medical:

- Prostaglandins +/– mifepristone (anti-progesterone).

Surgical:

- Suction curettage.

Map 3.2. Miscarriage

Map 3.3. Molar pregnancies

What is a molar pregnancy?

Molar pregnancies, also known as gestational trophoblastic disease, are due to excessive uncontrolled proliferation of trophoblastic tissue. They may be characterized as either partial or complete molar pregnancies and further characterized as benign or malignant.

Type of molar pregnancy	Benign or malignant?
Hydatidiform mole	Benign
Invasive mole	Malignant
Choriocarcinoma	Malignant

Causes

- Partial moles are made from both maternal and paternal genetic material.
- Complete moles are made from only paternal genetic material.

Risk factors

- Extremes of maternal age.
- More common in women of Asian ancestry.

Symptoms

- Uterus large for dates.
- Vaginal bleeding.
- Hyperemesis.
- Rare symptoms: pre-eclampsia, hyperthyroidism.

Investigations

- β-hCG levels: excessively high.
- Blood pressure.
- Blood tests: FBC, U&E, TFTs (group and save, rhesus status if excessive bleeding).
- Radiology: transvaginal USS – a 'snow storm' appearance is pathognomonic.

MAP 3.3. **Molar pregnancies**

Complications

- Increased risk of trophoblastic disease in subsequent pregnancies.
- Trophoblastic disease may become persistent and require chemotherapy.
- Choriocarcinoma may metastasize.

Treatment

Conservative:
- Patient education.
- Contact specialist centres for trophoblastic disease.

Medical:
- Prostaglandins +/– mifepristone (anti-progesterone) sometimes used to aid removal of trophoblastic tissue.
- Chemotherapy may be required.

Surgical:
- Suction curettage.

Table 3.1. Sexually transmitted infections

TABLE 3.1. **Sexually transmitted infections.**

Disease	Causative organism	Symptoms	Investigations	Treatment
Chlamydia	*Chlamydia trachomatis*	• Asymptomatic (there is currently an opportunistic screening programme in the UK for under 25's) • Females: vaginal discharge, inter-menstrual or post-coital bleeding, cervicitis • Males: urethritis, dysuria • It is the most common cause of pelvic inflammatory disease	Nucleic acid amplification test (NAAT) from either endocervical swabs/urine sample for women and a urine sample for men	• Doxycycline (7 days) • Azithromycin (single dose)
Trichomoniasis	*Trichomonas vaginalis*	• Asymptomatic • Females: vaginal discharge (green and offensive), vulvovaginitis, 'strawberry cervix', superficial dyspareunia, pH >4.5 • Males: urethritis	Wet mount microscopy to visualize motile trophozoites	• Metronidazole
Gonorrhoea	*Neisseria gonorrhoeae*	• Females: generally asymptomatic, vaginal discharge, cervicitis • Males: urethritis	Endocervical swabs	• azithromycin and IM ceftriaxone
Genital warts (condylomata accuminata)	Human papillomavirus (HPV)	• Papilliform or flat warts • May be pigmented • May bleed • May itch	Clinical presentation	• First line – topical podophyllum or cryotherapy • Second line – imiquimod cream

Genital herpes	Herpes simplex virus (HSV) 1 and 2	• Painful, ulcerated lesions • Dysuria • Lymphadenopathy	Viral swab	• Aciclovir
Syphilis	*Treponema pallidum*	See Map 2.12 (p. 58) Split into: • Primary syphilis – chancre • Secondary syphilis – rash • Tertiary syphilis – cardiac and neurological involvement. Gummata formation	See Map 2.12 (p. 58) VDRL testing	• Penicillin

Table 3.1 Sexually transmitted infections

Table 3.2. Non-sexually transmitted infections

TABLE 3.2. **Non-sexually transmitted infections.**

Disease	Causative organism	Symptoms	Investigations	Treatment
Candidiasis	*Candida albicans*	• Typical discharge ('cottage cheese') • Itching • Vulvitis	• Microscopy and culture	• Topical preparations (e.g. imidazoles) • Oral preparations (e.g. fluconazole)
Bacterial vaginosis	*Gardherella vaginalis*	• May be asymptomatic • Amsel's criteria – three of the four criteria listed below must be met: 1. White homogeneous discharge 2. Clue cells visible on microscopy 3. Vaginal pH >4.5 4. Positive whiff test – a fishy odour is created on addition of potassium hydroxide	• Refer to Amsel's criteria: microscopy, increased vaginal pH, addition of potassium hydroxide	• Oral metronidazole (5–7 days) • Second line – topical metronidazole or clindamycin

TABLE 3.3. **Menorrhagia. In layman's terms, menorrhagia is heavy menstrual bleeding. Previously it was defined objectively as >80 mL blood loss; however, there has been a shift to the subjective where heavy menstrual bleeding is defined by what the woman feels is excessive.**

Causes	Investigations	Treatment
Remember as **U BLEED**: U – Uterine polyps/Uterine fibroids B – **Bleeding disorders** (e.g. von Willebrand disease) L – Likely no underlying pathology (50%) E – Endometriosis E – Endometrial carcinoma/hyperplasia D – pelvic inflammatory Disease/intrauterine Devices	Depends on the cause of menorrhagia. It is essential to perform an FBC in each case to exclude anaemia. Some investigations are listed below: • General blood tests: FBC, U&E, TFTs • Radiology: USS, hysteroscopy, endometrial biopsy if indicated Refer to appropriate local algorithms.	Treatment is a stepwise approach. **Medical:** • First-line: Mirena intrauterine system • Second-line: mefenamic acid (particularly if co-morbid dysmenorrhoea), tranexamic acid, combined oral contraceptive pill • Third-line: long acting progestogens (oral or injected). Consider GnRH analogues if this fails **Surgical:** • Endometrial ablation • Hysterectomy • **Note:** Surgical intervention can cause infertility

Table 3.3. Menorrhagia

What is amenorrhoea?

This may be defined as either primary or secondary amenorrhoea:

- Primary: menstruation has not commenced by the age of 16.
- Secondary: the absence of menstruation for 6 months in a woman who previously had normal menstruation.

Causes

These are split into primary and secondary causes.

Primary causes (2T 2C):

- Turner syndrome (45,X).
- Testicular feminization.
- Congenital malformations (e.g. Mayer–Rokitansky–Küster–Hauser syndrome [Müllerian agenesis], imperforate hymen).
- Congenital adrenal hyperplasia.

Symptoms

Depends on the cause of amenorrhoea. Some examples are listed below:

- Polycystic ovary syndrome (see Map 3.5, p. 84).
- Turner syndrome – webbed neck, short stature.
- Premature ovarian failure – associated with other autoimmune conditions such as Addison's disease and hypothyroidism.
- Mayer–Rokitansky–Küster–Hauser syndrome – varying degrees of uterovaginal aplasia or hypoplasia.

Investigations

- β-hCG levels (urine or serum) to exclude pregnancy.
- Blood tests: FBC, U&E, TFTs, gonadotropin levels, prolactin levels, androgen levels, oestradiol.
- Radiology: may be required to visualize suspected tumours if clinically indicated.

MAP 3.4. Amenorrhoea

Map 3.4. Amenorrhoea

Secondary causes (4P 3H):

- Pregnancy – the most common cause.
- Polycystic ovary syndrome (see Map 3.5, p. 84).
- Premature ovarian failure.
- Pituitary necrosis – Sheehan's syndrome after PPH.
- Hyperprolactinaemia.
- Hypothalamic disorder (e.g. anorexia nervosa, excessive exercise, stress).
- Hyper/Hypothyroidism.

Treatment

Depends on the cause of amenorrhoea. Some examples are listed below.

Conservative:

- Patient education.

Medical:

- Polycystic ovary syndrome (see Map 3.5, p. 84).
- Premature ovarian failure – hormone replacement therapy.

Surgical:

- Depends on underlying pathology (e.g. Mayer–Rokitansky–Küster–Hauser syndrome – the use of vaginal dilators and surgical procedures such as the Vecchietti procedure.

Complications

- Infertility.
- Osteoporosis.

Map 3.4. Amenorrhoea

Map 3.5. Polycystic ovary syndrome (PCOS)

What is polycystic ovary syndrome?

This is when a woman has polycystic ovaries. It is diagnosed using the Rotherham criteria where two out of the three criteria listed below must be met:

1. Radiological features: a USS visualizing multiple (>12) small follicles measuring ~2–9 mm +/– an ovarian volume >10 mL.
2. Menstrual irregularity: periods that are >5 weeks apart.
3. Endocrine phenomena:
   - Hyperandrogenism – hirsutism, acne.

Causes

The exact cause of PCOS is unknown. Factors include insulin resistance and hormonal imbalance causing increased androgen levels, decreased levels of sex hormone binding globulin (SHBG), raised LH levels and sometimes raised prolactin levels.

Symptoms

May be asymptomatic but other features may be remembered as **HAIR:**

H – Hirsutism
A – Amenorrhoea
I – Irregular periods/Increased weight
R – Reduced fertility and miscarriage

Investigations

- General blood tests: FBC, U&E, TFTs.
- Specific blood tests: androgen levels, SHBG, LH, FSH, prolactin.
- Radiology: transvaginal USS for specific features (see Rotherham criteria).

MAP 3.5. **Polycystic ovary syndrome (PCOS)**

Treatment

Conservative:

- Patient education.
- Lifestyle advice – particularly weight loss.

Medical: this aims to treat symptoms

- Hirsutism: oral contraceptive pills with an antiandrogen effect (e.g. Yasmin or Dianette).
- Subfertility: metformin may help.
- Inducing ovulation: clomifene.

Surgical:

- Not indicated. IVF may be required later.

Complications

- Infertility.
- Type 2 diabetes mellitus.
- Gestational diabetes.
- Depression.
- Increased weight, which leads to complications such as:
  - ○ Sleep apnoea.
  - ○ Metabolic syndrome.
  - ○ Increased risk of diabetes.
  - ○ High blood pressure.

Map 3.5. Polycystic ovary syndrome (PCOS)

TABLE 3.4. Termination of pregnancy (TOP).

Current legal standing	Methods used	Complications

Based on the Abortion Act 1967; amended 1990 by the Human Fertilization and Embryology Act. Requires the signatures of two registered practitioners. Full details of the Human Fertilization and Embryology Act may be found at: http://www.legislation.gov.uk/ukpga/1990/37/contents
 	
Key features of the Act:
 	
• Must be no greater than 24 weeks gestation
• May be considered >24 weeks gestation if the life of the mother is at great risk
• Consider in cases where there may be great risk to the mother's existing children
• Consider when the physical or mental health of the mother is in great jeopardy
• Consider if the child is highly likely to be born with a severe mental or physical handicap
	The method used for TOP depends on the gestation of the pregnancy. Generally, the methods used are as follows.
	
	1. <9 weeks gestation:
	  ○ Mifepristone
	  ○ 48 hours after dose of mifepristone give prostaglandin (e.g. misoprostol). Prostaglandins stimulate uterine contraction
	2. <13 weeks gestation:
	  ○ Surgical dilatation and vacuum aspiration
	3. 15 weeks gestation:
	  ○ Surgical dilatation and evacuation
		General complications:
		
		• Those of general anaesthetic
		• Haemorrhage
		• Infection
		• Retained products of conception
		• Psychiatric complications (e.g. depression)
		
		Specific complications:
		
		• Trauma to the genital tract
		• Asherman's syndrome
		• Perforation of pelvic organs (i.e. uterus, bowel and bladder)

Table 3.4. Termination of pregnancy (TOP)

Map 3.6. Infertility

What is infertility?

Infertility is the failure to conceive after regular unprotected intercourse for 2 years in the absence of known reproductive pathology. This may be categorized as being either primary or secondary. In the former the couple have never conceived, whereas in secondary infertility the couple has previously conceived.

Fertility requires a normal sperm to reach a normal egg and then fertilize it. This fertilized egg then needs to implant successfully into the endometrium. Any hindrance in this process may cause infertility.

Causes

These are classified into male and female causes. Some examples are listed below:

- **Male:** occurs when there is a problem with sperm volume, pH, concentration, morphology, motility or vitality. This may be due to smoking, alcohol use, steroids or STIs.
- **Female:** think of the hypothalamic ovarian axis to remember the causes:
  - Hypothalamic dysfunction:
    - Hyperprolactinaemia.
    - Hypothalamic hypogonadism.
    - Hypothyroidism.
    - Hyperthyroidism.

Symptoms

- Primary or secondary infertility.
- Those of underlying cause.

Investigations

- Semen analysis. Normal results are:
  - Volume >1.5 mL.
  - pH >7.2.
  - Sperm concentration >15 million/mL.
  - Morphology >4% normal forms.
  - Motility >32% progressive motility.
  - Vitality >58% live spermatozoa.
- Blood tests: FBC, U&E, TFTs, androgen levels, SHBG, LH, FSH, prolactin, 21-day progesterone (>30 nmol/L = ovulation).
- Radiology: transvaginal USS, hysterosalpingogram.
- Laparoscopy and dye tests.

Map 3.6. Infertility

- ○ Ovarian dysfunction:
  - – PCOS.
  - – Premature ovarian failure.
- ○ Tubal dysfunction:
  - – PID.
  - – Adhesions from previous pelvic surgery.
  - – Cystic fibrosis.
- ○ Implantation failure:
  - – Fibroids.
- ○ Anatomical abnormality:
  - – Bicornate uterus.
  - – Mayer–Rokitansky–Küster–Hauser syndrome.

Treatment

Depends on the cause of infertility.

Conservative:
- Patient education.
- Regular intercourse 3–4 times a week.
- Lifestyle advice – particularly weight loss.

Medical:
- Clomifene.
- Gonadotropin therapy.

Surgical:
- Ovarian diathermy.
- IVF.
- Intra-uterine insemination.
- Tubal surgery.

Complications

- Psychological implications – depression and anxiety.
- Side effects of treatments including:
  - ○ Ovarian hyperstimulation syndrome.
  - ○ Ectopic pregnancy.
  - ○ Multiple pregnancy.

Map 3.7. Cervical cancer

What is cervical cancer?

This is uncontrolled differentiation and proliferation of cells lining the cervix. It may be categorized into two different cell types:

1. Squamous cell carcinoma (80%).
2. Adenocarcinoma (20%).

Causes

The exact cause of cervical cancer remains unknown but it is associated with several risk factors, the most prominent being the human papillomavirus (HPV) (see below).

Risk factors

- HPV – types 16, 18 and 33.
- HIV.
- Multiple pregnancies.
- Multiple sexual partners.
- Early age of first sexual intercourse.
- Combined oral contraceptive pill (COCP).
- Increasing age.
- Low socioeconomic status.
- Smoking.

Symptoms

- Intermenstrual bleeding.
- Post-coital bleeding.
- Post-menopausal bleeding.
- Abnormal vaginal discharge.
- General symptoms of malignancy (e.g. fatigue, cachexia, weight loss).
- Asymptomatic – abnormalities picked up by the National Screening Programme (NSP) UK. The NSP for cervical cancer uses liquid-based cytology to classify cervical intraepithelial neoplasia as well as identify HPV infection. This occurs 3 yearly aged 25–49 and 5 yearly aged 50–64, providing that results are normal.

Investigations

- General blood tests: FBC, U&E, LFTs, TFTs.
- Specific blood tests: colposcopy with biopsy of cervix.
- Radiology: MRI of pelvis.
- Stage using the Fédération Internationale de Gynécologie et d'Obstétrique (FIGO) system.

MAP 3.7. **Cervical cancer**

Cervical ectropion

Does not cause cervical cancer but is included in the differential diagnosis of vaginal bleeding.

What is cervical ectropion?

This is when a greater proportion of columnar epithelium crosses the transition zone and is present on the ectocervix rather than stratified squamous cell epithelium. Columnar epithelium is thinner and far more fragile than stratified squamous cell epithelium, therefore it is more prone to bleeding.

Causes: anything that increases oestrogen levels (e.g. COCP, pregnancy).

Symptoms: post-coital bleeding, abnormal vaginal bleeding, bleeding on contact (e.g. at colposcopy).

Treatment: ablative cold coagulation.

Treatment

Depends on FIGO stage and whether or not metastases are present.

Conservative:
- Patient education.
- Lifestyle advice – smoking cessation.
- Prevention (UK): HPV vaccination offered to schoolgirls aged 12.

Medical:
- Chemotherapy and radiotherapy may be required.

Surgical:
- Cone biopsy.
- Hysterectomy.

Complications

- Psychological implications – depression and anxiety.
- General and specific complications of chemotherapy and radiotherapy.
- Lymphoedema if lymph nodes are removed.
- Fistula formation.
- Metastases.
- Death.

Map 3.8: Vaginal cancer

What is vaginal cancer?

This is uncontrolled differentiation and proliferation of cells lining the vagina. It may be categorized into different cell types:

- Squamous cell carcinoma (most common).
- Adenocarcinoma.
- Clear cell adenocarcinoma.
- Germ cell tumours (e.g. teratomas).
- Melanoma.

Causes

The exact cause of vaginal cancer remains unknown but it is associated with several risk factors (see below).

Risk factors

Remember these as **VAGINA**:

V – **V**iruses (e.g. HPV, HIV)

A – increasing **A**ge

G – **G**eneral factors such as smoking and alcohol

I – chronic **I**rritation (e.g. from prolonged pessary use)

N – **N**eoplasms (e.g. having cervical cancer increases the risk of vaginal squamous cell carcinoma)

A – vaginal **A**denosis

Symptoms

- Asymptomatic.
- Intermenstrual bleeding.
- Post-coital bleeding.
- Post-menopausal bleeding.
- Abnormal vaginal discharge.
- Dyspareunia.
- General symptoms of malignancy (e.g. fatigue, cachexia, weight loss)

Investigations

- General blood tests: FBC, U&E, LFTs, TFTs.
- Specific blood tests: colposcopy with biopsy.
- Radiology: MRI pelvis.
- Stage using the FIGO system or the TNM staging system.

MAP 3.8. **Vaginal cancer**

Complications

- Psychological implications – depression and anxiety.
- General and specific complications of chemotherapy and radiotherapy.
- Lymphoedema if lymph nodes are removed.
- Fistula formation.
- Metastases.
- Death.

Treatment

Depends on FIGO stage and whether or not metastases are present.

Conservative:

- Patient education.
- Lifestyle advice – smoking cessation.
- Prevention (UK): HPV vaccination offered to schoolgirls aged 12.

Medical:

- Chemotherapy and radiotherapy may be required.

Surgical:

- Partial or radical vaginectomy.
- Radical vaginectomy plus radical hysterectomy.
- Pelvic exenteration.

Map 3.8. Vaginal cancer

Map 3.9: Endometrial cancer

What is endometrial cancer?

This is uncontrolled differentiation and proliferation of the endometrium.

It may be categorized into different cell types, most of which are adenocarcinomas.

Causes

It is due to the unopposed action of oestrogen on the endometrium. Risk factors are listed below.

Risk factors

Remember these as **ENDOMETRIUM:**

E – Early menarche

N – Nulliparity

D – Diabetes mellitus

O – polycystic **O**vary syndrome

M – Menopause (late)

E

T – Tamoxifen

R – HRT

I – Increased risk with other cancers (e.g. breast and ovarian)

U – Unopposed oestrogen (e.g. anovulation, HRT)

M – Menstrual irregularity

Symptoms

- A woman with post-menopausal bleeding is considered to have endometrial cancer until proven otherwise.
- Premenopausal women: intermenstrual bleeding, post-coital bleeding.
- General symptoms of malignancy (e.g. fatigue, cachexia, weight loss)

Investigations

- General blood tests: FBC, U&E, LFTs, TFTs.
- Radiology: first line – transvaginal USS (<4 mm = normal),
- This may be followed by hysteroscopy with endometrial biopsy.
- MRI of pelvis – for staging and metastases.
- Stage using the FIGO system or the TNM staging system.

Complications

- Psychological implications – depression and anxiety.
- General and specific complications of chemotherapy and radiotherapy.
- Lymphoedema if lymph nodes are removed.
- Fistula formation.
- Metastases.
- Death.

Treatment

Depends on FIGO stage and whether or not metastases are present.

Conservative:
- Patient education.

Medical:
- Chemotherapy and radiotherapy may be required.

Surgical:
- Total abdominal hysterectomy with bilateral salpingo-oophorectomy +/- lymphadenectomy.

Map 3.9. Endometrial cancer

Map 3.10. Ovarian cancer

What is ovarian cancer?

This is uncontrolled differentiation and proliferation of ovarian tissue. Approximately 90% arise from epithelial tissue. May occur secondarily (e.g. metastasis from another site, usually the GI tract, where it is known as a Krukenberg tumour).

Causes

The exact cause of ovarian cancer is unknown; however, it is strongly associated with multiple ovulations and other risk factors (see below).

Risk factors

Remember these as **ABCDE**:

A – increasing Age

B – *BRCA1* and *BRCA2* genes

C – COCP is protective!

D – Duration of ovulation (i.e. nulliparity, early menarche and late menopause)

E – Endometriosis

Symptoms

Symptoms are generally really vague, which is why ovarian cancer can be so difficult to diagnose. Symptoms include:

- Abdominal pain.
- Abdominal bloating.
- Intermenstrual bleeding.
- Post-coital bleeding.
- Early satiety.
- Symptoms of bladder dysfunction or irritation such as frequency and urgency.
- General symptoms of malignancy (e.g. fatigue, cachexia, weight loss).

Investigations

- General blood tests: FBC, U&E, LFTs, TFTs.
- Tumour marker: CA 125 (diagnosis and follow-up).
- Radiology: transvaginal USS.
- CT or MRI of pelvis – for staging and metastases.
- Surgery: diagnostic laparotomy with biopsy.
- Stage using the FIGO system or the TNM system.
- Risk of Malignancy Index (RMI) may be used to calculate the risk of having a malignant ovarian tumour = ultrasound score × menopausal score × CA 125 measurement.

MAP 3.10. Ovarian cancer

Complications
- Psychological implications – depression and anxiety.
- General and specific complications of chemotherapy and radiotherapy.
- Lymphoedema if lymph nodes are removed.
- Fistula formation.
- Metastases.
- Death.

Treatment
Depends on FIGO stage and whether or not metastases are present.

Conservative:
- Patient education.

Medical:
- Chemotherapy usually required and radiotherapy may be required.

Surgical:
- Depends on the individual case and may include oophorectomy, salpingectomy, hysterectomy, omentectomy.

Table 3.5. Ovarian cysts

TABLE 3.5. Ovarian cysts. Ovarian cysts may be benign or malignant. Ultrasound is used to assess which is more likely. Unilocular cysts are likely physiological/benign, whereas multilocular complex cysts raise suspicion of a malignant lesion.

Type of cyst	Key features
Follicular cyst	The most common type of physiological cyst
Corpus luteum cyst	Higher tendency to cause intraperitoneal bleeding
Dermoid cyst	Benign germ cell tumour Torsion more likely

Epithelial tumours	1. Serous cystadenoma:
	   ○ Commonest
	   ○ May mimic features of serous carcinoma
	2. Mucinous cystadenoma:
	   ○ May be massive in size

Endometrioma	Also known as 'chocolate cysts' Complication of endometriosis **What is endometriosis?** A condition where endometrial tissue occurs outside the uterine cavity. **Causes:** The exact cause is unknown but the present theory regards retrograde menstruation as the most likely factor. **Symptoms:** Chronic pelvic pain, retroverted uterus, dysmenorrhoea, deep dyspareunia. **Investigations:** Bimanual and speculum examination followed by laparoscopy. **Treatment:** • Conservative: patient education. • Medical: a stepwise approach is employed. First line: NSAIDs. Second line: paracetamol. Third line: codeine. Hormonal therapy such as the COCP may be used if these pain medications fail. • Surgical: laser ablation, adhesiolysis, total abdominal hysterectomy.

TABLE 3.6. **Incontinence.**

Type	What is it?	Investigations	Treatment
Stress incontinence	• Urine is lost by any movement that increases intra-abdominal pressure (e.g. sneezing and coughing) • Aggravating factors include pregnancy, obesity, COPD	• Urinalysis • Post-void residual volume • Urodynamic testing • Endoscope tests • Radiology: x-ray, USS	• Conservative: patient education, lifestyle advice such as smoking cessation, weight loss • First line: Kegel pelvic floor exercises • Medical: oestrogen may be given to post-menopausal women • Surgery: urethropexy, bladder neck suspension surgery (Burch and sling procedures)
Urge incontinence	• Too much contraction • Urine is lost by inappropriate detrusor muscle contraction • Cause: may be due to neoplasms or nerve damage (e.g. multiple sclerosis, Parkinson's disease, stroke)	• Urinalysis • Post-void residual volume • Urodynamic testing • Endoscope tests • Radiology: x-ray, USS	• Anticholinergic medications (e.g. oxybutynin therapy) • Treatment of underlying condition
Overflow incontinence	• Too little contraction • This happens due to a marked increased in bladder residual volume; therefore, the bladder is usually full and thus frequently leaks urine	• Urinalysis • Post-void residual volume • Urodynamic testing • Endoscope tests • Radiology: x-ray, USS	• Conservative: patient education, stop medications if they are the cause • Intermittent catheterization • Bethanechol (cholinergic) may improve detrusor muscle activity

Table 3.6. Incontinence

TABLE 3.7. **Contraception. Consult the UKMEC guidelines regarding contraceptive choices (http://www.fsrh.org/pdfs/UKMEC2009.pdf).**

Efficacy of contraception depends on the Pearl Index (the number of unintended pregnancies per 100 woman years).

A high Pearl Index equates to a higher chance of an unintended pregnancy.

Type	Examples
Barrier methods	Condom – male and female Diaphragm Cap
Hormonal contraception	COCP: • Mechanism of action: prevents ovulation and prevents implantation by thinning the endometrial lining • Many contraindications. Refer to UKMEC guidelines. There are four categories in the UKMEC guidelines; 1 – generally safe; 2 – benefits outweigh the risks; 3 – risks outweigh the benefits; 4 – unsafe • Effective contraception: after 7 days POP: • Mechanism of action: thickens the cervical mucus and secretions making it inhospitable to sperm • Effective contraception: after 2 days Contraceptive injection: • Depo-Provera is mainly used in the UK • Given 12 weekly • Delay in return of fertility once stopping the injection. Make take up to 12 months to return • Effective contraception: after 7 days

Intrauterine contraception	**Contraceptive implant:** • The radiopaque implant (Nexplanon) is inserted subdermally in the non-dominant arm • Is the long-acting contraception of choice in young people who may not reliably take the pill • Effective contraception: after 7 days **Emergency contraceptive pill:** • 1.5 mg levonorgestrel taken within 72 hours of unprotected intercourse **Intrauterine device (IUD):** • IUD also known as the copper coil • Mechanism of action: the copper ions are thought to create a hostile environment for sperm • Effective contraception: immediately **Interuterine system (IUS):** • IUS, also known as the Mirena system, releases levonorgestrel • Mechanism of action: thickens cervical mucus and secretions. Prevents endometrial proliferation • Effective contraception: after 7 days
Irreversible contraception	**Male sterilization:** • An easier procedure to perform than female sterilization • May be done as an outpatient procedure under local anaesthesia • Two semen samples must be supplied after the procedure at 16 and 20 weeks to ensure that it has worked **Female sterilization:** • Performed under general anaesthesia • Many different methods may be used (e.g. Filshie clips or Falope rings)

Table 3.7. Contraception

Map 4.1. Neonatal jaundice

What is neonatal jaundice?

Jaundice, also known as icterus, is the yellow discolouration of mucous membranes, sclera and skin. This occurs due to the accumulation of bilirubin. Jaundice may be seen at a bilirubin concentration >42.8 μmol/L (2.5 mg/dL).

Causes

The causes of jaundice may be split into three categories:
1. Pre-hepatic jaundice.
2. Intra-hepatic jaundice.
3. Post-hepatic jaundice.

For neonates it may be further subdivided into a time scale: <24 hours, 24 hours to 3 weeks, and >3 weeks. See Table opposite for more details.

Symptoms

Poor feeding, failure to thrive and yellow discolouration as well as **SICK**:

S – Seizures

I – Irritability, Increased muscle tone

C – Coma

K – Kernicterus

Treatment

Treat underlying cause

Complications

- Liver failure.
- Renal failure.
- Sepsis.
- Pancreatitis.
- Biliary cirrhosis.
- Cholangitis.

Investigations

Must determine underlying cause.

Use these tests to determine the type of jaundice:

- Appearance of urine and stool.
- LFTs.
- Bilirubin levels.
- Alkaline phosphatase levels.

Table to show the different blood results for different types of jaundice:

Investigation	Pre-hepatic jaundice	Intra-hepatic jaundice	Post-hepatic jaundice
Appearance of urine	Normal	Dark	Dark
Appearance of stool	Normal	Normal or pale	Pale
Conjugated bilirubin	Normal	↑	↑
Unconjugated bilirubin	Normal or ↑	↑	Normal
Total bilirubin	Normal or ↑	↑	↑
Alkaline phosphatase	Normal	↑	↑

MAP 4.1. Neonatal jaundice

Time elapsed postnatally	Cause

<24 hours	Infection (e.g. TORCHES [see Map 2.6, p. 50])
	 Haemolytic disorders:
	 • ABO incompatibility.
	 • Rhesus incompatibility.
	 • G6PD deficiency:
	   ○ X-linked condition.
	   ○ Deficiency in glucose-6-phosphate dehydrogenase. Resultant effect is a decrease in antioxidant NADPH meaning that RBCs are more susceptible to oxidative stress (e.g. infection/certain foods such as fava beans). Blood smear: Heinz bodies; bite cells.
	 • Spherocytosis:
	   ○ Autosomal dominant condition.
	   ○ Caused by functional abnormality of structural RBC membrane proteins (e.g. spectrin, ankyrin)
	   ○ Blood smear: spherocytes.

24 hours to 3 weeks	Remember as **ABC**: **A** – A physiological cause **B** – Breast milk jaundice **C** – Crigler–Najjar syndrome: autosomal recessive condition. Two types: type 1: absence of UDP glucuronosyl transferase 1-A1; type 2: reduced levels of UDP glucuronosyl transferase 1-A1. Haemolysis Infection
>3 weeks	Unconjugated causes: infection, a physiological cause, haemolytic causes. Conjugated causes: hepatitis, obstructed bile duct.

Map 4.1. Neonatal jaundice

Map 4.2. Necrotizing enterocolitis (NEC)

What is necrotizing enterocolitis?
This is an inflammatory bowel necrosis.

Causes
The exact cause of NEC is unknown, but the present theory concerning the pathophysiology of NEC involves a hypoxic insult that occurs in a premature infant because their immune system is not fully developed. Hypoxia occurs and this causes intestinal sloughing. This allows bacteria to invade the intestinal wall and cause inflammation. This eventually leads to gangrene, risk of perforation and NEC.

Investigations
- Blood tests: FBC, WCC, U&E (there may be a metabolic acidosis).
- Radiology: abdominal x-ray (pneumatosis intestinalis/perforation). May show other signs (e.g. football sign [massive pneumoperitoneum], thumbprinting [large bowel oedema]).

Symptoms
- Intolerant of feeds.
- Abdominal distension.
- Decreased bowel sounds.
- Bloody stools.
- Vomiting (may be bile stained).
- Shock.

MAP 4.2. **Necrotizing enterocolitis (NEC)**

Complications
- Death.
- Short bowel syndrome.
- Bowel obstruction.
- Anaemia.

Treatment

Conservative:
- Information provided to parents.
- Stop bottle feeding.
- Admit to NICU and take serial x-rays looking for perforation.
- Continually monitor girth measurement.

Medical: only consider if no perforation evident:
- Decompress the large bowel.
- Provide broad-spectrum antibiotics (check hospital guidelines).
- Intravenous fluids and nutrition.

Surgical:
- Manage surgically if perforated.

Map 4.2. Necrotizing enterocolitis (NEC)

Map 4.3. Hypertrophic pyloric stenosis

What is hypertrophic pyloric stenosis?
This is when the muscular layer of the pyloris hypertrophies, resulting in a gastric outlet obstruction by narrowing the outlet from the stomach to the duodenum. It presents around 2–8 weeks of age.

Causes
Hypertrophy of the muscular layer of the pyloris. The exact reason why this happens remains unclear but there are some associated risk factors (see below).

Risk factors (remember as the 3Fs):
First-born males
Family history of the disorder
Fair skin

Investigations
- Feeding test may show peristaltic wave.
- Blood tests: FBC, WCC, U&E, LFTs (there may be a hypochloraemic alkalosis).
- Monitor urine output.
- Radiology: USS confirms diagnosis

MAP 4.3. Hypertrophic pyloric stenosis

Symptoms
Remember as **PYLORIC**:
- **P** – Projective vomiting (non-bilious) worsening with time
- **Y** – Yelling, unhappy child
- **L** – Lethargic child, Loss of weight
- **O** – 'Olive' (pyloric mass) present in the RUQ
- **R** – Rumbling tummy (i.e. gastric peristalsis from left to right seen on feeding test)
- **I** – Irritable
- **C** – Constipated

Complications
- Electrolyte imbalances.
- Duodenal perforation.
- Apnoea.
- Aspiration pneumonia.

Treatment

Conservative:
- Parent education.
- Continual monitoring.

Medical:
- Correct electrolyte imbalance.

Surgical:
- Ramstedt's pyloromyotomy.

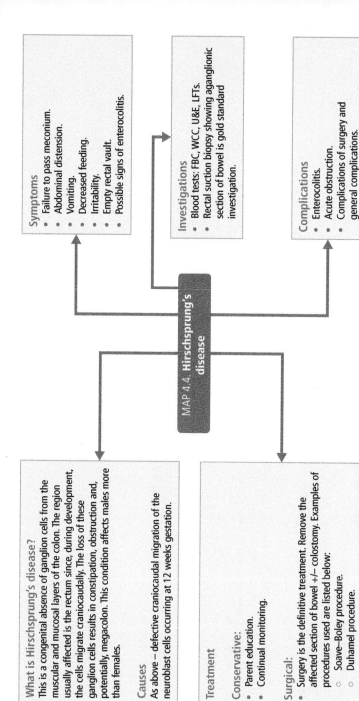

What is Hirschsprung's disease?

This is a congenital absence of ganglion cells from the muscular and mucosal layers of the colon. The region usually affected is the rectum since, during development, the cells migrate craniocaudally. The loss of these ganglion cells results in constipation, obstruction and, potentially, megacolon. This condition affects males more than females.

Causes

As above – defective craniocaudal migration of the neuroblast cells occurring at 12 weeks gestation.

Treatment

Conservative:
- Parent education.
- Continual monitoring.

Surgical:
- Surgery is the definitive treatment. Remove the affected section of bowel +/– colostomy. Examples of procedures used are listed below:
  ○ Soave–Boley procedure.
  ○ Duhamel procedure.

MAP 4.4. Hirschsprung's disease

Symptoms

- Failure to pass meconium.
- Abdominal distension.
- Vomiting.
- Decreased feeding.
- Irritability.
- Empty rectal vault.
- Possible signs of enterocolitis.

Investigations

- Blood tests: FBC, WCC, U&E, LFTs.
- Rectal suction biopsy showing aganglionic section of bowel is gold standard investigation.

Complications

- Enterocolitis.
- Acute obstruction.
- Complications of surgery and general complications.

What is intussusception?

This is when a portion of the intestine becomes invaginated into its own lumen to a variable degree by peristalsis.

Causes

These may be split into paediatric and adult causes.

Paediatric:
- Meckel's diverticulum. This is the remnant of the vitelline duct (joins yolk sac to the midgut lumen) that usually obliterates during 9th week of gestation. It is associated with the rule of **2s:**
  - It affects **2%** of the population.
  - **2 times** more common in males.
  - It is **2 inches** long.
  - It is located **2 feet** from the iliocaecal valve (although, in reality, this may be any distance).
  - It contains **2 types** of tissues, gastric and pancreatic, which is why a technetium-99m scan is the investigation of choice.
- Hypertrophied Peyer's patches

Adults
- Tumour.

Symptoms

Symptoms present in a classic triad:
1. Pain – severe, colicky abdominal pain.
2. Blood in stool – often described as 'redcurrant jelly'.
3. Vomiting – non-bilious initially but may become bilious.

MAP 4.5. Intussusception

Investigations

- Blood tests: FBC, WCC, U&E, LFTs (usually unremarkable blood results).
- Radiology: abdominal x-ray – may visualize dilated loops of bowel or perforation.
- USS – 'target sign'

Note: Air/contrast enema may be used as it is both diagnostic and therapeutic.

Treatment

Conservative:
- Parent education.
- Continual monitoring.

Radiological (see investigations section):
- Hydrostatic reduction using enema.

Surgical:
- May be required if other measures fail.

Complications

- Perforation.
- Shock.
- Peritonitis.

TABLE 4.1. Anterior abdominal wall defects. The differences between an omphalocoele and a gastroschisis are outlined below.

	Omphalocoele	Gastroschisis
Location	Midline defect. It is a ventral defect of the umbilical ring	Paraumbilical defect due to incomplete fusion of the abdominal wall
Covered by viscera	Yes	No
Associated with other defects	Yes. Generally, midline defects are associated with other abnormalities such as cardiac, genitourinary or chromosomal abnormalities	No. However, this condition has an association with cocaine use and babies who are small for gestational age
Investigations	Detected antenatally via sonography	Detected antenatally via sonography
Treatment	Several steps need to be followed: 1. The abdominal contents must be protected. This may be achieved using moistened, sterile gauze 2. Fluids and electrolytes must be monitored and corrected if necessary 3. The lesion must be closed (e.g. using a silo). This must be done slowly because if closed too quickly, the sudden addition of the abdominal contents may cause haemodynamic compromise and decrease venous return to the heart	Several steps need to be followed: 1. The abdominal contents must be protected. This may be achieved using moistened, sterile gauze 2. Fluids and electrolytes must be monitored and corrected if necessary 3. Provide broad-spectrum antibiotics. 4. Surgery is necessary usually within 24–48 hours

Table 4.1 Anterior abdominal wall defects

Map 4.6. Congenital cardiac defects

Atrial septal defects (ASDs):

Ostium primum:
- Caused by a failure of the septum primum to join the endocardial cushion.
- Associated with other neural crest migration defects since the endocardial cushion is primarily formed from neural crest cells that have migrated to the endocardial tube during embryological development.

Ostium secundum:
- Eight times more common than the primum type.
- Caused by excessive absorption of the septum primum or incomplete growth of the septum secundum.

Acyanotic defects

Type	Cause	Features
Tetralogy of Fallot	Dextraposition of the aorticopulmonary septum (aka the spiral septum)	Remember as **PROV**: P – Pulmonary stenosis R – Right ventricular hypertrophy O – Overriding aorta V – VSD
Persistent truncus arteriosis	The spiral septum fails to form	A VSD forms since the spiral septum is the source of the membranous intraventricular septum
Transposition of the great vessels	During development the aorticopulmonary septum spirals through a 180 degree anticlockwise rotation, hence its name the spiral septum. This places the great vessels into their appropriate anatomical position (i.e. the aorta posterior and to the right, the pulmonary trunk anterior and to the left). In this condition the aorticopulmonary septum fails to spiral	Associated with other defects that allow the shunting of blood, otherwise the neonate would die

MAP 4.6. **Congenital cardiac defects**

What are congenital cardiac defects?

This is when the heart fails to develop normally. They may be broadly categorized as cyanotic and acyanotic.

Cyanotic defects: right → left shunt

- Truncus arteriosus.
- Transposition of the great vessels.
- Tricuspid insufficiency.
- Tetralogy of Fallot.

Acyanotic defects: left → right shunt

- Remember as the 3Ds:
  VSD – most common defect
  ASD
  PDA

Causes

Depends on the specific defect, but there are many risk factors associated with them:

- Unknown.
- Maternal factors: e.g. TORCHES infection (see Map 2.6, p. 50), diabetes mellitus and systemic lupus erythematosus.
- Teratogens:
  ○ Alcohol.
  ○ Lithium.
  ○ Warfarin.
  ○ Phenytoin.
- Chromosomal abnormalities.

Murmurs

Condition	Murmur	Location best heard
VSD	Pansystolic. Smaller lesions are loudest	Lower left sternal edge
ASD	Systolic ejection	Upper left sternal edge
PDA	Machinery murmur	Upper left sternal edge
Tetralogy of Fallot	Systolic ejection	Upper left sternal edge
Transposition of the great vessels	No murmur	N/A

Map 4.6. Congenital cardiac defects

Horseshoe kidney

What is a horseshoe kidney?

This occurs during development when the upper and lower poles of the kidneys fuse and cannot ascend to their normal anatomical position due to the inferior mesenteric artery. This results in a horseshoe shape.

Causes: congenital abnormality.

Signs and symptoms:
- Asymptomatic.
- Recurrent urinary tract infections.
- Renal calculi.
- Obstructive uropathy.

Investigations: USS is diagnostic.

Treatment: treatment of complications.

Complications:
- Susceptible to trauma.
- Renal calculi formation.
- Increased risk of transitional cell carcinoma of the renal pelvis.

Genitourinary abnormalities are associated with **CHARGE:**

C – **C**oloboma
H – **H**eart defects
A – **A**tresia of the nasal choanae
R – **R**etarded growth/development
G – **G**enitourinary abnormalities
E – **E**ar abnormalities/deafness

Autosomal recessive polycystic kidney disease

What is autosomal recessive polycystic kidney disease (ARPKD)?

This is a recessively inherited polycystic disease found in children.

Causes:
- *PKHD1* on chromosome 6.

Signs and symptoms:
- Hypertension.
- Those of chronic kidney injury.
- Chronic respiratory infections.
- Those of portal hypertension: ascites, caput medusae and oesophageal varices (vomiting blood).
- Failure to thrive.
- Recurrent urinary tract infections.
- Polyuria.

Investigations: antenatal screening is diagnostic. Shows enlarged kidney with or without oligohydramnios.

Treatment: no specific treatment. Manage hypertension. Dialysis and kidney transplantation should be considered. Long-term oxygen therapy is often required due to chronic respiratory infections.

Complications:
- Hepatic cysts.
- Congenital hepatic fibrosis.
- Proliferative bile ducts.

MAP 4.7. **Genitourinary abnormalities**

Bladder exstrophy

What is bladder exstrophy?
This is a congenital malformation where the bladder protrudes through an abdominal wall defect.

Causes: congenital abnormality.

Signs and symptoms: remember as **ABCDES**:
A – Abdominal wall defect
B – Boys also have epispadias
C – Clitoris is bifid in girls affected
D – Divergent labia may also be present
E – Externally rotated pelvis
S – Shortened pubic rami

Investigations: clinical diagnosis aided with USS.

Treatment: surgery.

Complications:
- Vesicoureteral reflux (diagnosed after a micturating cystourethrogram).
- Urinary tract infections.
- Bladder spasm.

Hypospadias

What is hypospadias?
This is a congenital malformation of the urethral groove, meaning that the urethral opening occurs on the ventral aspect of the penis. The hypospadias is classified by the location of the urethral opening. Epispadias is when the urethral opening occurs on the dorsal aspect of the penis.

Causes: congenital abnormality.

Signs and symptoms:
Classic triad of:
1. Abnormal urethral opening.
2. Chordee (bend of penis).
3. Hooded foreskin.

Investigations: clinical diagnosis.

Treatment: surgery.

Complications:
- Infection.
- Haematoma.
- Fistula.
- Stenosis.

Map 4.7. Genitourinary abnormalities

Table 4.2. Neurocutaneous syndromes

TABLE 4.2. **Neurocutaneous syndromes.**

Condition	Genetics	Notes
Neurofibromatosis	Autosomal dominant Type 1: neurofibromin defect chromosome 17q11 Type 2: merlin defect chromosome 22q12	Type 1: • Aka von Recklinghausen disease • Skin manifestations: ○ Café au lait spots ○ Axillary freckling ○ Neurofibromas ○ Lisch nodules (hamartomas on the iris) • Increased risk of optic glioma Type 2: • Skin manifestations are more mild than type 1 • Associated with acoustic neuromas and deafness
Tuberous sclerosis	Autosomal dominant Type 1: hamartin defect chromosome 9 Type 2: tuberin defect chromosome 16	Skin manifestations: ○ Ash leaf spots ○ Shagreen patches ○ Adenoma sebaceum • Associated with epilepsy and benign tumours
Hereditary haemorrhagic telangiectasia	Autosomal dominant condition Most due to mutations of: • *ENG* chromosome 9 • *ACVRL1* chromosome 12	• Aka Osler–Weber–Rendu syndrome • Associated with telangiectasia, epistaxis and vascular disorders of the central nervous syndrome

| Sturge–Weber syndrome | Mutation of the *GNAQ* gene causes abnormality of mesoderm and ectoderm development | • Skin manifestation: facial port wine stain
• Radiological appearance: intracranial lesions and typical tram track calcifications
• Associated with epilepsy, hemiplegia, glaucoma and mental retardation |

Table 4.2. Neurocutaneous syndromes

Map 4.8. Neural tube defects (NTDs)

What are neural tube defects?

These are congenital abnormalities in the development of the spine, spinal cord and brain. They occur to varying degrees but the most common is spina bifida, a disorder in which the spinal column does not completely close.

Causes

The exact cause of NTDs is not known. However, they are associated with teratogens such as antiepileptic medication, maternal diabetes mellitus and high maternal BMI.

Investigations

- Antenatally on ultrasound.
- Triple marker test at 16–18 weeks:
  1. Alpha fetoprotein levels (α-FP).
  2. Oestriol levels (uE3).
  3. Human chorionic gonadotropin (hCG).

Condition	α-FP	uE3	hCG
Spina bifida	↑	Normal	Normal
Anencephaly	↓	↓	↓

Symptoms

Vary depending on type of NTD. A brief outline is provided below:

- Anencephaly: the brain and cranium fail to develop resulting in fetal death.
- Encephalocoele: aka cranium bifidum. This is a condition where the brain, covered by its meninges, protrudes through a midline cranial defect.
- Spina bifida: this occurs when the spinal column or vertebral arch fails to close. The spinal column may be tethered, which leads to problems with bladder control. On examination, there is often hair overlying the defect.
- Meningocoele: is associated with spina bifida. The meninges protrude through the defect but it does not contain the spinal cord.
- Meningomyelocoele: is associated with spina bifida. The meninges and spinal cord protrude through the defect.

MAP 4.8. Neural tube defects (NTDs)

Treatment

Depends on the type of NTD.

Conservative:
- Parent education.
- Folic acid supplementation – higher dose to mothers at risk (e.g. those taking antiepileptic medication).
- Braces, crutches and other walking aids to help child's mobility.

Medical:
- Treatment of symptoms (e.g. UTIs and difficulty with bladder control).

Surgical:
- Release tethered cord.
- Shunts for hydrocephalus.
- Closure if spinal cord exposed.

Complications
- Decreased bladder control.
- Increased risk of UTI.
- Decreased mobility.
- Learning difficulties.
- Hydrocephalus.
- Complications of surgery and general anaesthetic.

Map 4.8. Neural tube defects (NTDs)

Map 4.9. Cerebral palsy

What is cerebral palsy?

This is a non-progressive insult that occurs on the developing brain. It results in a disorder of movement and posture as well as other neurological complaints such as epilepsy, depending on the location of the lesion.

Causes

There are many different causes of cerebral palsy including:

- Infection – meningitis and TORCHES.
- Trauma – in early childhood years or at birth.
- Hypoxia.
- Prematurity – increases risk.
- Vascular malformation (e.g. arteriovenous malformations, stroke).
- Tumours.

Symptoms

The symptoms depend on the subtype of cerebral palsy (remember as **SAD**). Split symptoms into:

1. Motor abnormality.

Subtype	Notes
Spastic	Most common ~80% Scissoring posture since flexors, adductors and internal rotators are largely affected Patient may present with diplegia, hemiplegia or quadriplegia
Ataxic	Abnormal sense of body in space
Dyskinetic	Abnormal, involuntary posturing

2. Learning difficulties.
3. Neurological abnormalities: patients may suffer with epilepsy.
4. Behavioural abnormalities: disordered sleep and self-injurious behaviour.
5. Sensory impairment: visual impairment including refractory errors as well as strabismus. Increased risk of deafness. Essential to screen for both.
6. Pseudobulbar palsy: present in some patients. Affects speech and swallowing.

MAP 4.9. Cerebral palsy

Investigations

Generally this is a clinical diagnosis, but identifying the cause may be aided by radiological investigation such as CT and MRI. It is also important to perform an audiological assessment as well as an ophthalmological evaluation.

Complications

- Orthopaedic complications: muscle shortening, abnormal posturing.
- Neurological complications: epilepsy.
- Respiratory complications: aspiration pneumonia, restrictive lung disease.
- Gastrointestinal complications: gastro-oesophageal reflux disease, constipation.
- Urinary complications: UTI, bladder control issues.
- Dermatological complications: decubitus ulcers.
- Psychological complications: depression.
- Sleep disorders.
- Learning difficulties.

Treatment

Conservative:
- Parent and patient education.
- Access to support services.

Medical:
- Manage complications.
- Antiepileptic medication.
- Others such as benzodiazepines and baclofen may be required.

Surgical:
- Muscle lengthening.
- Orthopaedic surgery (e.g. spinal fusion).
- Selective dorsal rhizotomy.

Map 4.9. Cerebral palsy

Map 4.10. Meningitis

What is meningitis?

This is an infection of the subarachnoid space by an organism that subsequently causes inflammation of the meninges.

Causes

There are many different causes of meningitis (see below).

Category	Age affected	Organisms
Bacterial	Neonate to 2 months	Group B streptococcus *Escherichia coli* *Listeria monocytogenes*
	1 month to 6 years	*Neisseria meningitidis* *Streptococcus pneumoniae* *Haemophilus influenzae* type B

Symptoms

- General symptoms:
  - Lethargy.
  - Crying.
  - Off feeds.
- Signs of increased intracranial pressure:
  - Decreased level of consciousness.
  - Papilloedema.
  - Headache.
- Specific signs:
  - Purpuric non-blanching rash (*Neisseria meningitidis*).
  - Neck stiffness.
  - Kernig's sign.
  - Focal neurological signs (e.g. cranial nerve involvement).

Investigations

- Blood tests: FBC, WCC, U&E, LFTs, glucose, group and save, clotting studies, blood cultures and PCR for *N. meningitidis*.
- General investigations: throat swab, urinalysis microscopy and culture, stool sample.
- Lumbar puncture: contraindicated if raised intracranial pressure or meningococcal septicaemia. Values shown below. PCR required for viral diagnosis.

Organism	WCC	Protein	Glucose
Bacterial	Neutrophils	↑	↓
Viral	Lymphocytes	Normal	Normal

- Radiology: CT if indicated.

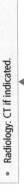

MAP 4.10. **Meningitis**

	Over 6 years	*Neisseria meningitidis* *Streptococcus pneumoniae* Mumps
	Any age	*Mycobacterium tuberculosis*
Viral	Any age	Enterovirus Cytomegalovirus Arbovirus

Risk factors: remember as **ABCS:**

A – Age (young)
B – Being of low socioeconomic status
C – Complement defects
S – Sickle cell disease

Treatment

Conservative:
- Parent education.
- Contact public health consultant since it is a notifiable disease.

Medical:
- GP may give IM benzylpenicillin in their practice to prevent delay.
- IV antibiotics depend on age:
  - <3 months: amoxicillin and cefotaxime.
  - >3 months: cefotaxime.
- Dexamethasone if >1 month and causative organism is *Haemophilus influenzae*.
- Antibiotic prophylaxis for close meningococcal contacts with rifampicin.

Complications

Meningitis causes several complications. Some are listed below.
Remember as the **5Cs:**

C – Cerebral palsy
C – Convulsions
C – Circulatory shock
C – Cerebral abscess
C – Cranial nerve palsies

Map 4.10. Meningitis

Map 4.11. Failure to thrive

What is failure to thrive?

This is when the child's weight or rate of weight gain is significantly less than their identically matched peers.

Causes

There are many causes of failure to thrive, which may be congenital or acquired. Some are categorized below:

- Not enough dietary intake:
  - Abuse and neglect.
  - Anorexia nervosa.
  - Poor parental dietary understanding.
- Difficulty feeding:
  - Cleft palate.
  - Oesophageal atresia/tracheo-oesophageal atresia.
  - Neurological disorders (e.g. cerebral palsy).
- Malabsorption:
  - Coeliac disease.
  - Inflammatory bowel disease (IBD).
  - Lactose intolerance.
- Chronic disease:
  - Cystic fibrosis.
  - Asthma.
  - Growth hormone deficiency.
  - Hypothyroidism.
- Chromosomal abnormalities:
  - Turner syndrome.
- Genetic abnormalities:
  - Achondroplasia.
  - Inborn errors of metabolism.

Symptoms

- General symptoms:
  - Lethargy.
  - Decreased weight.
  - Off feeds.
- Signs and symptoms of underlying disease (see below):

Condition	Notes
Anorexia nervosa	See Map 1.6 (p. 22)
Cerebral palsy	See Map 4.9 (p. 120)
Cystic fibrosis	See Map 4.14 (p. 130)
Asthma	See Map 4.15 (p. 132)
Abuse	Bruising of varying age. Changing history not in keeping with injuries
Hypothyroidism	Cold intolerance, constipation, dry skin/hair, hyporeflexia, bradycardia
Achondroplasia	Autosomal dominant inheritance. A cause of dwarfism. Due to mutation of fibroblast growth factor receptor 3 (FGFR3)
Coeliac disease	Proximal small intestine mainly affected. Associated with other autoimmune conditions and dermatitis herpetiformis

MAP 4.11. Failure to thrive

Investigations

- Blood tests: FBC, U&E, LFTs, TFTs, glucose.
- Urinalysis.
- Stool microscopy and culture.
- Specific test (e.g. sweat test for cystic fibrosis, endomesial and gliadin antibodies for coeliac disease).
- Chromosomal analysis if indicated.
- Radiology: may be required in certain circumstances (e.g. cerebral palsy may require CT or MRI).

Complications

- Psychological issues (e.g. depression).
- Decreased growth.
- Developmental delay.
- Specific problems related to cause.

Treatment

Conservative:
- Parent education.
- Involve social workers if necessary.
- Ensure child has an appropriate diet and is receiving the necessary calories.

Medical:
- Treat the underlying cause.

Surgical:
- If indicated.

Map 4.11. Failure to thrive

Map 4.12. Bronchiolitis

What is bronchiolitis?

This is a lower respiratory tract infection that is characterized by progressive symptoms from coryza to a persistent cough, breathlessness and possible respiratory distress. This condition often affects children <1 year of age since their airways are so narrow.

Causes

Remember as **RIP**:

R – Respiratory syncytial virus (most common cause)

I – Influenza

P – Parainfluenza

Symptoms

- General symptoms:
  - Breathlessness.
  - Persistent cough.
  - Lethargy.
  - Off feeds.
- Signs of respiratory depression:
  - Nasal flaring.
  - Subcostal and intercostal recession.
  - Low Glascow Coma Scale score.
  - Cyanosis.
- Signs of hyperinflation:
  - Downward displacement of liver.
- On auscultation:
  - Expiratory wheeze.
  - Fine end inspiratory crackles.

Investigations

- Blood tests: FBC, U&E, LFTs.
- Capillary blood gas.
- Specific tests: nasal aspirates with immuno-fluorescent staining for respiratory syncytial virus.
- Radiology: chest x-ray

**MAP 4.12.
Bronchiolitis**

Treatment

Conservative:
- Parent education.
- Continual monitoring.
- High-risk infants may require prophylactic palivizumab (e.g. infants who are premature or have congenital heart defects).

Medical:
- Humidified oxygen delivered via a nasal cannula.
- Ventilation required if symptoms are severe.
- Bronchodilators may be used but their benefit is unproven.

Complications
- Ventilation may be required (this may increase the risk of pneumonia).
- Respiratory failure.
- Cardiac failure.
- Pneumothorax.

Map 4.12. Bronchiolitis

Map 4.13. Croup

What is croup?

This is a viral infection that causes progressive inflammation of the respiratory tract commencing with the larynx and spreading distally to the bronchi. This is why it is also known as acute laryngotracheobronchitis. Tends to affect children aged 6 months to 6 years.

Causes

Remember as **RIP**:

R – Respiratory syncytial virus

I – Influenza

P – Parainfluenza (most common cause)

Symptoms

Tends to be worse at night

- **General symptoms:**
  ○ Breathlessness.
  ○ Persistent cough.
  ○ Lethargy.
  ○ Off feeds.
- **Typical features:** worsen with progression of inflammation:
  ○ Coryza +/– fever (prodrome).
  ○ 'Barking' cough.
  ○ Hoarseness.
  ○ Stridor.
- **Signs of respiratory depression:**
  ○ Nasal flaring.
  ○ Subcostal and intercostal recession.
  ○ Low Glasgow Coma Scale score.
  ○ Cyanosis.
- **On auscultation:**
  ○ Stridor – heard in moderated croup with a stethoscope. It is possible to hear stridor without a stethoscope in severe cases.

Investigations

- Blood tests and an examination of the child's throat is usually not undertaken since this may distress the child and inadvertently close their airway, leading to an emergency situation in which invasive access to the airway must be established.
- Heart rate, respiratory rate and oxygen saturation.
- Assess severity using the Westley Croup Score:

Category	Westley score	Features
Mild	0–2	Occasional cough. No stridor. No signs of respiratory depression
Moderate	3–5	Frequent cough. Stridor. Sternal wall retraction at rest
Severe	6–11	Frequent cough. Marked stridor. Marked sternal wall retraction. Respiratory distress

MAP 4.13. **Croup**

Treatment
Depends on the severity of croup.

Conservative:
- Parent education.
- Continual monitoring.

Medical:

Mild	Most may be managed at home with paracetamol, new guidance recommends giving a single dose of oral dexamethasone to all children regardless of severity.
Moderate	Steroids, e.g.: - Oral dexamethasone or prednisolone - Nebulized budesonide
Severe	1. Steroids, e.g.: - Oral dexamethasone or prednisolone - Nebulized budesonide 2. Nebulized adrenaline (5 mL of 1:1,000 with oxygen)

Complications
- Death.
- Tracheitis.
- Pneumonia.

Map 4.14 Cystic fibrosis (CF)

What is cystic fibrosis?

This is an autosomal recessive condition that occurs in 1 in 2,500 live births and has a carrier rate of 1 in 25. It occurs due to a deletion in phenylalanine, meaning that an abnormal cystic fibrosis transmembrane conductance regulator (CFTR) protein is then created. This in turn decreases Cl^- ion transport resulting in thickened dehydrated secretions.

Causes

It is caused by a deletion in phenylalanine, most commonly at position 508 on chromosome 7.

Symptoms

Symptoms and how the disease manifests itself may vary depending on the age of the child.

Neonate:
- Meconium ileus.

Young child:
- Failure to thrive.
- Frequent chest infections.
- Steatorrhoea.
- Signs of clubbing commence.

Older child:
- Frequent chest infections.
- Asthma.
- Allergic bronchopulmonary aspergillosis.
- Steatorrhoea.

Adulthood:
- As above.
- Bronchiectasis.
- Infertility.
- Diabetes.
- Cor pulmonale.
- Depression.
- Cirrhosis.

MAP 4.14.
Cystic fibrosis (CF)

Investigations
Depend on age of patient and when the disease presents.
- Specific tests:
  ○ Newborn blood spot: immunoreactive trypsinogen (IRT)
  ○ Sweat test:
    – Cl⁻ >50 mmol/L
    – Na⁺ >60 mmol/L
- Blood tests with every acute exacerbation: FBC, U&E, LFTs.
- Identify cause of infection using sputum analysis, chest x-ray and blood culture. Common organisms include *Staphylococcus aureus*, *Haemophilus influenzae*, *Pseudomonas aeruginosa*.
- Radiology:
  ○ Chest x-ray:
    – Bronchiectasis: 'tram tracks'.
    – Consolidation.
    – Fibrosis.

Treatment

Conservative:
- Parent education (e.g. keep children with CF separate to avoid cross-infection).
- Continual monitoring with multidisciplinary team involvement.
- Up to date immunizations.
- Physiotherapy (e.g. Flutter®, a mucus clearance device used by respiratory physiotherapists).

Medical:
- Treat infections according to cultural sensitivities. Consult microbiology and hospital guidelines. Some examples are given below:
  ○ Piperacillin in combination with tazobactam.
  ○ Tobramycin.
  ○ Meropenem.
  ○ Imipenem.
- Pancreatic enzyme supplements (e.g. Creon).
- Fat soluble vitamins.

Complications
- Increased frequency of respiratory tract infections.
- Bronchiectasis.
- Respiratory failure.
- Infertility.
- Diabetes.
- Gallstones.
- Cor pulmonale.
- Malnutrition.
- Nasal polyps.
- Depression.

Map 4.14 Cystic fibrosis (CF)

Map 4.15. Asthma

What is asthma?

Asthma is a chronic, inflammatory disease that is characterized by reversible airway obstruction.

In children it affects boys more than girls, but in adults, females are more greatly affected.

Causes

The cause of asthma is multifactorial encompassing both genetic and environmental elements:

- **Genetic:**
  - Personal/family history of atopy – involvement of chromosome 11.
  - Family history of asthma.
- **Environmental:**
  - Indoor allergens:
    - House dust mite.
    - Pets.
    - Fungal spores.
  - Outdoor allergens:
    - Pollen.
    - Cold air.

Symptoms

- Respiratory features: wheeze, cough, shortness of breath.
- Symptoms worse at night or early morning.
- Symptoms may occur after exercise or a triggering factor such as cold weather.
- Symptoms may occur after beta blockers.
- Decreased peak expiratory flow rate (PEFR) and forced expiratory volume in 1 second.
- Personal/family history of asthma/atopy.
- Unexplained blood eosinophilia.

Investigations

- Blood tests: FBC, U&E, LFTs, eosinophils.
- Sputum sample if indicated.
- Pulmonary function tests:
  - PEFR: diurnal variation.
  - Spirometry: $FEV_1/FVC <0.7$ (obstructive defect).
- Radiology:
  - Chest x-ray: only if required/in acute setting. May show pneumothorax or consolidation.

MAP 4.15. **Asthma**

- Occupational allergens:
  - Isocyanates.
  - Epoxyresins.
  - Other factors:
    - Smoking.
    - Infection.
    - Emotion.
    - Drugs (e.g. beta blockers).

The above triggering factors cause the classic triad that characterizes asthma:
1. Copious mucus secretion.
2. Inflammation of the airways.
3. Contraction of bronchial smooth muscle.

This triad occurs due to the activation of Th2 cells, which upregulate the immune response. Th2 cells stimulate the release of the following:
- Interleukin (IL)-4: stimulates eosinophils and B lymphocytes.
- IL-5: stimulates eosinophils.
- IL-13: stimulates mucus production.

Treatment

Conservative:
- Patient education.
- Advice on inhaler technique, use of spacer devices and avoidance of triggering factors.
- Annual asthma review and influenza vaccine required.

Medical:
- Refer to British Thoracic Society Guidelines (see Table 4.3, p. 134).

Complications

- Death.
- Disturbed sleep.
- Persistent cough.
- Side effects of steroids, e.g.:
  - Weight gain.
  - Thinning of the skin.
  - Striae formation.
  - Cataracts.
  - Cushing's syndrome.
  - Growth disturbance.

Table 4.3. Flow chart summarizing the British Thoracic Society guidelines

TABLE 4.3. **Flow chart summarizing the British Thoracic Society guidelines.**
https://www.brit-thoracic.org.uk/document-library/clinical-information/asthma/btssign-asthma-guideline-quick-reference-guide-2014/

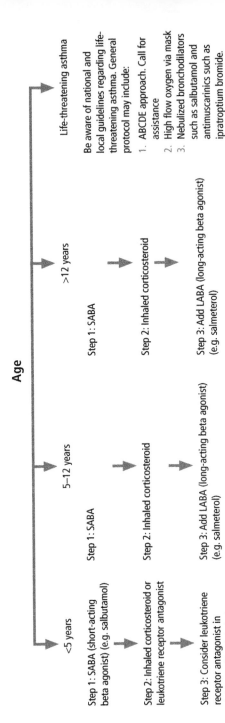

Age

<5 years

Step 1: SABA (short-acting beta agonist) (e.g. salbutamol)

Step 2: Inhaled corticosteroid or leukotriene receptor antagonist

Step 3: Consider leukotriene receptor antagonist in children taking inhaled steroid. Consider inhaled steroid in children already taking leukotriene receptor antagonist

5–12 years

Step 1: SABA

Step 2: Inhaled corticosteroid

Step 3: Add LABA (long-acting beta agonist) (e.g. salmeterol)

Assess control:

- If well controlled: continue regime
- If partial improvement: continue regime but increase inhaled corticosteroid dose

>12 years

Step 1: SABA

Step 2: Inhaled corticosteroid

Step 3: Add LABA (long-acting beta agonist) (e.g. salmeterol)

Assess control:

- If well controlled: continue regime
- If partial improvement: continue regime but increase inhaled corticosteroid dose

Life-threatening asthma

Be aware of national and local guidelines regarding life-threatening asthma. General protocol may include:

1. ABCDE approach. Call for assistance
2. High flow oxygen via mask
3. Nebulized bronchodilators such as salbutamol and antimuscarinics such as ipratropium bromide. Monitor response.
4. Secure IV access and consider hydrocortisone
5. Further methods should be initiated under specialist supervision and include aminophylline bolus or magnesium sulphate IV

Step 4: Refer to specialist

Step 4: Increase inhaled corticosteroid dose

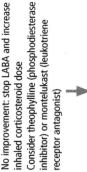

Step 5:
* Steroid tablet (prednisolone)
* Highest dose inhaled corticosteroid
* Refer to specialist

* No improvement: stop LABA and increase inhaled corticosteroid dose
* Consider theophylline (phosphodiesterase inhibitor) or montelukast (leukotriene receptor antagonist)

Step 4:
* Increase inhaled corticosteroid dose
* Consider theophylline (phosphodiesterase inhibitor), montelukast (leukotriene receptor antagonist) or beta 2 agonist tablet

Step 5:
* Steroid tablet (prednisolone)
* Highest dose inhaled corticosteroid
* Refer to specialist

* No improvement: stop LABA and increase inhaled corticosteroid dose
* Consider theophylline (phosphodiesterase inhibitor) or montelukast (leukotriene receptor antagonist)

Table 4.3 Flow chart summarizing the British Thoracic Society guidelines

Map 4.16. Rheumatic fever

What is rheumatic fever?

Rheumatic fever is a rare inflammatory disorder that is now more common in those from the Asian subcontinent. Tends to affect children aged 5–15 years old.

Causes

- Group A beta haemolytic streptococcus (e.g. *Streptococcus pyogenes*).
- Rheumatic fever is preceded by a streptococcal pharyngitis and then affects all layers of the heart, creating a pathological lesion called an Aschoff body.
- Other regions of the body as well as the heart are affected, such as the skin, central nervous system and the musculoskeletal system.

Symptoms

Diagnosed using the Jones criteria: 2 major or 1 major and 1 minor criteria PLUS a preceding streptococcal throat infection.

Remember major criteria as **ABCD**:

A – **A**rthritis (polyarthritis)
B – **B**eating heart (carditis)
C – Syndenham's **C**horea
D – **D**ermatological manifestations (e.g. subcutaneous nodules and erythema marginatum)

Remember minor criteria as **FAT PAD**:

F – **F**ever
A – **A**rthralgia
T – **T**hroat swab positive for Group A beta haemolytic *Streptococcus*
P – **P**revious rheumatic fever/prolonged PR interval
A – **A**cute phase reactants (e.g. CRP/ESR/leucocytosis)
D – **D**/A

MAP 4.16. **Rheumatic fever**

Investigations

- Throat swabs.
- Blood tests: FBC, U&E, LFTs, ASO titres or DNAase.
- ECG: prolonged PR interval.
- ECHO: visualize heart valve affected.

Treatment

Conservative:
- Patient and parent education.

Medical:
- Aspirin is the initial treatment of choice for inflammation but is contraindicated in children due to Reye syndrome, which is a rapidly progressive encephalopathy.
- Corticosteroids may be used for inflammation.
- Antibiotics (e.g. penicillin). Check sensitivities with microbiology and hospital guidelines.

Complications

- Chronic rheumatic heart disease: mitral valve affected in 50%.
- Atrial fibrillation.
- Heart failure.
- Predisposition for infective endocarditis.

Map 4.16. Rheumatic fever

Map 4.17. Urinary tract infection (UTI)

What is a urinary tract infection?

This is an infection of the urinary tract with typical signs and symptoms. It may be classified as either lower or upper (acute pyelonephritis).

In children, UTIs are more common in boys until the age of 3 months. After this time the incidence is higher in girls.

Causes

UTIs are generally caused by infection of the urinary tract with *Escherichia coli*. However, there are several risk factors that may predispose to infection (see below).

Risk factors

- Female gender.
- Genitourinary malformations.
- Vesicoureteric reflux (VUR).
- Diabetes.
- Immunosuppression.
- Conditions that predispose to stone formation and therefore urinary tract obstruction.
- Catheterization.

Investigations

- Urine dipstick: positive for leucocytes and nitrites. The problem in paediatrics is collecting the urine sample and the method varies depending on the age of the child. Some examples include: clean catch method, collection pads and suprapubic aspiration.
  Urine culture: >10^5 organisms per mL of midstream urine.
- Radiology:
  ○ Kidneys, ureter and bladder USS for anatomical abnormalities.
  ○ Vesicoureteric reflux: micturating cystourethrogram.
  ○ Renal scarring: dimercaptosuccinic acid scan.

Symptoms

Generally depend on the age of the child.

Neonates:
- Off feeds.
- Irritable
- Foul smelling urine

Young children:
- Fever.
- Dysuria.
- Suprapubic pain.

Older children (more like adult symptoms):
- Fever.
- Dysuria.
- Frequency.
- Urgency.
- Suprapubic pain.

Upper UTI:
- Fever/chills.
- Flank pain.
- Haematuria.

MAP 4.17. **Urinary tract infection (UTI)**

Treatment

Conservative:
- Parent and patient education.

Medical:
- Depends on the age of the child and type of infection.
- Treat according to cultural sensitivities after contacting microbiology and consulting local guidelines.

Age	Action
<3 months	Refer
>3 months with lower UTI	Antibiotics (e.g. trimethoprim or nitrofurantoin)
>3 months with upper UTI	Admit and antibiotics (e.g. co-amoxiclav)

Complications
- Pyelonephritis.
- Hydronephrosis.
- Renal failure.
- Renal abscess.
- Sepsis.

Map 4.18. Haemolytic uraemic syndrome (HUS)

What is haemolytic uraemic syndrome?
This is a syndrome that predominantly affects children.

Causes
Usually *Escherichia coli* O157:H7 or *Shigella* enteritis. These organisms enter the body via contaminated food or water. Then they express viratoxins, which cause damage by binding to glomerular endothelial cells, resulting in renal insufficiency, destroying red blood cells and causing anaemia and platelet damage.

Symptoms
HUS is comprised of a triad. Remember as **MAT**:
1. **M** – Microangiopathic haemolytic anaemia
2. **A** – Acute kidney injury
3. **T** – Thrombocytopenia

Other symptoms include:
● Nausea
● Vomiting
● Bloody diarrhoea
● Abdominal pain
● NO FEVER

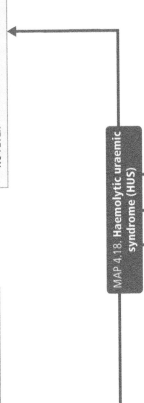

MAP 4.18: Haemolytic uraemic syndrome (HUS)

Investigations

- Stool culture.
- Urinalysis and estimated GFR.
- Blood tests: FBC, U&E, LFTs, Cr:BUN, LDH.
- Peripheral blood smear: schistocytes.

Treatment

Conservative:

- Involve the nephrologists and haemotologists
- HUS is a notifiable disease in the UK.
- Patient and parent education.
- Monitor BP.

Medical:

- Treatment is generally supportive.
- Hydrate patient with IV fluids.
- If hypertension present, then consider calcium channel blockers.
- Consider dialysis and RBC transfusion if needed.

Complications

Remember as **ABCS**:

A – Acute kidney injury
B – increased **B**lood pressure
C – **C**hronic kidney injury
C – **C**ardiac complications (e.g. heart failure)
C – **C**oma
S – **S**troke

Map 4.18 Haemolytic uraemic syndrome (HUS)

Map 4.19. Henoch–Schönlein purpura (HSP)

What is Henoch–Schönlein purpura?

This is a systemic vasculitis that presents with typical signs and symptoms.

Causes

HSP is caused by IgA complex deposition in the capillaries, arterioles and venules in organs such as the skin and the kidneys, which causes symptoms via the activation of complement.

**MAP 4.19.
Henoch–Schönlein
purpura (HSP)**

Symptoms

HSP is comprised of a triad. Remember as **RAP:**

1. **R – Renal manifestations:**
   - Haematuria – microscopic/macroscopic.
   - ANCA negative glomerulonephritis.
   - Nephrotic syndrome (rare).
2. **A – Arthralgia and abdominal pain.**
3. **P – Purpura:**
   - This typically affects the buttocks and the lower limbs. However, it may affect the arms.

Investigations

- Urinalysis and estimated GFR.
- Blood tests: FBC, U&E, LFTs, Cr:BUN, LDH, CRP, ESR.
- IgA levels.
- Skin biopsy if indicated or if there is diagnostic uncertainty: immunofluorescence shows IgA deposits and C3.

Treatment

Conservative:
- Patient and parent education.

Medical:
- Treatment is generally supportive due to high rates of spontaneous remission.
- Analgesia.
- Steroids may sometimes be used in severe cases.

Complications
Remember as **ABC**:
- **A** – Acute kidney injury
- **B** – Bowel obstruction: intussusception
- **C** – Chronic kidney injury

Map 4.19 Henoch-Schönlein purpura (HSP)

Table 4.4. Childhood epilepsy syndromes

TABLE 4.4. **Childhood epilepsy syndromes.**

Type of epilepsy	Features	Investigations	Treatment
Absence	Cause: exact cause is unknown but is thought to involve T-type Ca^{2+} channels. Seizures may be triggered by hyperventilation Features: • Aka petit mal seizures • Consciousness is impaired • Often picked up as day dreaming in school • More common females • May be associated with automatisms (e.g. lip smacking)	EEG: 3Hz spike and wave	Ethosuximide
Benign rolandic epilepsy	Cause: unknown Features: • Occurs at night time • Abnormal sensation (e.g. paraesthesia of the corner of the patient's mouth and tongue) • Drooling and bed wetting may occur • Tends to remit by puberty	EEG: centrotemporal spikes	Often not used since the condition is benign Antiepileptics: carbamazepine is used first line

Lennox–Gastaut syndrome	Cause: overall the cause is unknown but it may occur secondary to congenital or acquired causes. Congenital causes include tuberous sclerosis and inherited metabolic disorders. Acquired causes include infection, trauma and tumours Features: • Varying types of seizures • Status epilepticus may occur • Associated with drop attacks • Associated with learning difficulties and developmental delay • Persists into adult life	EEG: Slow spike and wave	Difficult to treat Antiepileptic: sodium valproate is often used first line Prednisolone is sometimes used

West's syndrome	Cause: exact cause is unknown. However, there are theories that suggest the involvement of abnormal GABA neurotransmitter or the excessive production of corticotropin-releasing hormone
	
	Features:
	• There are three different types of attack:
	  1. Lightning attacks
	  2. Nodding attacks
	  3. Jackknife attacks
	• Associated with: ABCD:
	  A – Aicardi syndrome
	  B – Brain damage
	  C – Cerebral atrophy
	  D – Dysplasia of the corex
		EEG: hypsarrhythmia	Difficult to treat
			Antiepileptic: vigabatrin is often used first line
			Prednisolone is sometimes used

Table 4.4 Childhood epilepsy syndromes

What is diabetic ketoacidosis?

This is an emergency that is associated with type 1 diabetes (see Map 2.2, p. 40). It is a state of uncontrolled catabolism in which ketone bodies are formed. The ketone bodies are acetone, acetoacetate and beta-hydroxybutyrate. This may be the patient's first presentation to emergency services prior to a diabetic diagnosis or it may be brought on by the patient missing their insulin dose or because of stress (e.g. illness)

Causes

- Non-deliberate omission of insulin (e.g. illness).
- Deliberate omission of insulin (e.g. children with unstable family circumstances, co-morbid psychiatric disorder such as eating disorders or depression, psychosocial impact of having a chronic illness resulting in missed doses at school or university).

The pathophysiology of DKA is summarized in Figure 4.1 (p. 148).

Investigations

- Bloods: glucose levels, U&E, blood gases.
- Urinalysis: for ketones.
- If infection suspected, then obtain cultures (blood, urine, throat) and perform the 'septic six'.
- ECG – tented T-waves and broadening of the QRS complex may be seen in hyperkalaemia associated with potassium therapy
- ABG: assess the degree of acidosis.
- Amylase: abdominal pain and vomiting is also associated with pancreatitis.
- Radiology: chest x-ray may be required to locate source of infection.

Symptoms

General symptoms:

- Polyuria/enuresis.
- Polydipsia.
- Weight loss.
- Abdominal pain.
- Lethargy.
- Vomiting.
- Confusion.

Clinical signs of DKA:

- Dehydration.
- Polyuria.
- Polydipsia.
- Tachycardia.
- Hypotension.
- Kaussmaul breathing (to exhale excessive CO_2).
- Acetone sweet smelling breath.
- Confusion.
- Coma.

Biochemical signs:

- Ketonuria.
- Increased blood glucose level.
- Acidaemia.

MAP 4.20. **Diabetic ketoacidosis (DKA)**

Complications

- Coma.
- Complications of treatment, e.g.:
  - Cerebral oedema.
  - Hypokalaemia.
  - Hypoglycaemia.

Treatment

Resuscitation:

- Airway – +/– nasogastric tube.
- Breathing – 100% oxygen.
- Circulation – IV saline solution.

Clinically acidotic but not in shock:

- IV therapy – saline solution and additional KCl therapy (monitor ECG).
- Fixed rate insulin infusion of 0.1unit/kg/h IV (typically 50 units Actrapid® in 50ml 0.9% saline).
- Constant patient observations (e.g. glucose levels, urine output, fluid input, neurological status, electrolytes and ECG).
- Start broad-spectrum antibiotics if infection suspected.

Clinically well and tolerating oral fluids:

- Start subcutaneous insulin.
- Continue oral hydration therapy.

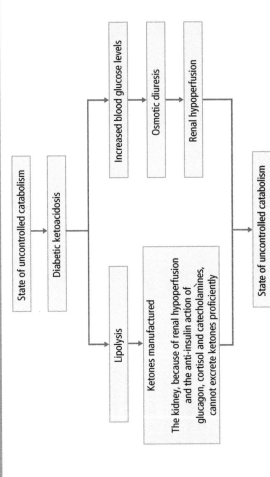

FIGURE 4.1. Pathophysiology of diabetic ketoacidosis

TABLE 4.5. **Trisomies.**

Trisomy	Syndrome name	Symptoms	Investigations	Complications
21	Down's syndrome	• Learning difficulties • Short stature • Flattened nose • Slanted eyes • Simian crease • Gap between 1st and 2nd toe	Antenatal testing – USS for nuchal translucency (see Table 2.1, p. 34) Radiology – pelvic x-ray shows dysplastic pelvis	• Atrial septal defects • Ventricular septal defects • Duodenal atresia • Acute lymphoblastic leukaemia • Alzheimer's disease • Hypothyroidism
18	Edward's syndrome	• Rocker bottom feet • Learning difficulties • Clenched hands • Low set ears • Micrognathia • Cleft lip or cleft palate • Undescended testicles	Chromosomal analysis confirms diagnosis ECG and ECHO – for cardiac complications	• Coarctation of the aorta • Atrial septal defects • Inguinal hernia • Omphalocoele • Renal agenesis
13	Patau's syndrome	• Learning difficulties • Congenital heart disease • Cleft lip/palate • Microcephaly • Polydactyly • Rocker bottom feet	Chromosomal analysis confirms diagnosis ECG and ECHO – for cardiac complications	• Omphalocoele • Polycystic kidneys • Ventricular septal defects • Inguinal hernia

Table 4.5. Trisomies

Map 4.21. Kawasaki's disease

What is Kawasaki's disease?
This is a rare form of autoimmune vasculitis; also known as lymph node syndrome. It is vital to diagnose due to its severe complications.

Causes
Exact cause is not known. It is thought to be an autoimmune vasculitis.

Symptoms
Remember as **ABCDES**:
A – A high fever >5 days
B – Bright red lips
C – Cervical lymphadenopathy
D – Desquamation of hands and feet
E – Eyes: non-purulent bilateral conjunctivitis
S – Strawberry tongue

Investigations
Kawasaki's disease is a clinical diagnosis and there is no specific test; however, it is vital to perform an ECHO looking for coronary aneurysms, which are a serious complication.

- Blood tests: FBC, WCC, U&E, LFTs, ESR, CRP.
- Urinalysis.
- ECG.
- Radiology:
  - ECHO.
  - USS/CT if indicated: may show gallbladder enlargement.

MAP 4.21. **Kawasaki's disease**

Complications

- Coronary aneurysms.
- Dysrhythmias.
- Myocarditis.
- Valvular abnormalities.

Treatment

Conservative:
- Patient and parent education.

Medical:
- IV immunoglobulin therapy.
- Aspirin (Kawasaki's disease is the only exception for the use of aspirin in children due to the risk of Reye syndrome).

Map 4.21. Kawasaki's disease

Table 4.6. Childhood cancers

TABLE 4.6. **Childhood cancers.**

Disease	Cause	Symptoms	Investigations	Treatment	Complications
Acute lymphoblastic leukaemia (ALL)	A rare neoplasm of the blood/bone marrow. The exact cause is unknown but it is likely due to a genetic susceptibility coupled with an environmental trigger. It is the commonest cancer in children. Associated with Down's syndrome	Bone marrow failure Bruising Shortness of breath Purpura Malaise Weight loss Night sweats	Bloods: FBC, WCC, platelets, U&E, LFTs, ESR, CRP Bone marrow biopsy, lymph node biopsy Radiology: x-ray, USS, CT, MRI ALL is classified using the French–American–British (FAB) classification	**To induce remission:** • Dexamethasone • Vincristine • Anthracycline antibiotics • Cyclophosphamide **Maintenance:** • Methotrexate • Mercaptopurine • Cytarabine • Hydrocortisone	• Death • Often spreads to the central nervous system • Increased risk of infection • Haemorrhage • Depression • Complications of chemotherapy
Neuroblastoma	This is a neuroendocrine tumour arising from neuroblast cells within the sympathetic nervous system. Neuroblastomas mostly originate in the adrenal glands but may develop anywhere along the sympathetic nervous system.	Symptoms differ depending on the location of the lesion. General symptoms: • Weight loss • Anorexia • Emesis	Bloods: FBC, WCC, platelets, U&E, LFTs, TFTs, ESR, CRP, calcium, magnesium, phosphorus, uric acid, LDH, IgG levels	Treatment depends on the stage of the tumour and is delivered by a multidisciplinary team.	• Relapse and recurrent disease • Metastasis

It is the most common extracranial solid tumour of infancy. The exact cause of neuroblastoma is unknown but *ALK* mutations have been identified in familial cases. Fifty to 60% present with metastases	Abdomen: • Abdominal pain • Swelling Chest: • Respiratory difficulty Bone/bone marrow: • Bone pain • Limp Paraspinal cord ganglia results in neurological symptoms such as: • Weakness • Paralysis • Bladder dysfunction • Bowel dysfunction Rare symptoms: • Hypertension (renal artery compression) • Chronic diarrhoea (vasoactive intestinal peptide secretion)	Increased levels of urine catecholamines (or their metabolites [e.g. homovanillic acid/vanillylmandelic acid]) Radiology: CT, meta-iodobenzylguanidine scan Histology: Homer Wright rosettes. Neuroblastomas are classified using the International Neuroblastoma Staging System (INSS)	**Medical:** common chemotherapy combinations include: • Vincristine, cyclophosphamide and doxorubicin • Cisplatin and etoposide • Carboplatin and etoposide • Ifosfamide and etoposide • Cyclophosphamide and topotecan **Surgical:** • Surgical resection in localized disease is curative • Surgery post chemotherapy may be seen as a debulking procedure	• Paraneoplastic syndromes (e.g. opsoclonus myoclonus syndrome) • Complications of chemotherapy

Continued overleaf

Table 4.6. Childhood cancers

Table 4.6. Childhood cancers

TABLE 4.6. **Childhood cancers** (*continued*).

Disease	Cause	Symptoms	Investigations	Treatment	Complications
Wilms' tumour (aka nephroblastoma)	Is a form of renal cancer that occurs in children. It is associated with aniridia. Nephroblastomas are mostly unilateral. It is associated with *WT1* gene mutations (chromosome 11p13) in 20% of cases. Syndromes associated with Wilms' tumours: • Denys–Drash syndrome • Frasier syndrome • Sporadic aniridia • Li-Fraumeni syndrome	• Abdominal swelling • Abdominal pain • Haematuria • Nausea • Vomiting	Bloods: FBC, WCC, platelets, U&E, LFTs, ESR, CRP, BUN Urinalysis Radiology: abdominal USS, abdominal x-ray, chest x-ray, CT abdomen, MRI, IV pyelogram	Treatment depends on the stage and size of the tumour as well as histopathological and molecular tumour features. **Chemotherapy:** some standard chemotherapy regimens are listed below: • Vincristine and dactinomycin • Vincristine, dactinomycin and doxorubicin • Vincristine, doxorubicin, cyclophosphamide and etoposide **Radiotherapy** **Surgical:** nephrectomy	• Metastasis • Hypertension, particularly if bilateral renal involvement

| Ewing's sarcoma | This is a rare, malignant small, round, blue cell tumour affecting the bone/soft tissue. It typically affects teenagers and young adults. Usually a result of t (11;22) translocations resulting in a *EWSR1/FLI1* fusion gene. The most common regions affected are:

• Pelvis
• Femur
• Humerus
• Ribs
• Clavicle | • Pain in the location of the tumour, which worsens over time
• A swelling in the location of the tumour
• Swelling and decreased range of movement of the affected joint
• Fever of unknown origin
• Unprovoked bone fracture
• General symptoms such as lethargy and weight loss | Bloods: FBC, WCC, platelets, U&E, LFTs, TFTs, ESR, CRP
Radiology: x-rays (show 'moth-eaten' radiolucencies), CT, MRI, PET, bone scintigraphy
Histology: small, round, blue cell tumour. Clear cytoplasm with H&E staining | Treatment depends on the stage and size of the tumour as well as histopathological features.

Chemotherapy: some chemotherapy regimens are listed below:

• Ifosfamide and etoposide
• Vincristine, doxorubicin and cyclophosphamide

Radiotherapy
Surgical: limb amputation | • Metastasis
• Limb amputation |

Table 4.6 Childhood cancers

Table 5.1: Sudden painless visual loss

TABLE 5.1. **Sudden painless visual loss.**

There are many causes of painless loss of vision. They may be remembered by the mnemonic OIROV:

Optical – occlusion of the retinal vein; Issues – ischaemic optic neuropathy; Really – retinal detachment; Obscure – occlusion of the retinal artery. Vision – vitreous haemorrhage.

Disease	Cause	Features	Investigations	Treatment
Occlusion of the retinal vein	• Hypertension • Glaucoma • Polycythaemia	• Sudden painless monocular vision loss or dense central scotoma • Ischaemic subtype is associated with acute presentation, whereas non-ischaemic subtype may present more subtly	• Visual acuity • Pupil analysis: may show an ipsilateral afferent pupillary defect • Intraocular pressure (IOP): usually normal • Anterior slit lamp examination: normal • Fundoscopy: diagnostic. Visualizes retinal haemorrhage and oedema (aka 'blood and thunder fundus') • Fluorescein angiography: retinal capillary ischaemia, macular oedema, neovascularization	Emergency care **Medical:** • No exact treatment. Manage risk factors and complications as they occur • Macular oedema: intravitreal anti-VEGF or steroids • Neovascularization: laser photocoagulation **Surgical:** • Vitrectomy

Ischaemic optic neuropathy	• Temporal arteritis
	• Atherosclerosis
	• Non-modifiable risk factors: age, male gender, positive family history
	• Modifiable risk factors: diabetes mellitus, hypertension, smoking, obesity, lipid and cholesterol levels
		• Visual loss: usually on waking
		• Temporal arteritis:
		  ○ General symptoms: weight loss, muscle aches (associated with polymyalgia rheumatica), scalp tenderness, temporal artery is thickened, tender but non pulsatile, jaw claudication
		  ○ Visual symptoms: optic neuropathy, blindness, diplopia
		  ○ Neurology symptoms: stroke, myelopathy, neuropathy
			• Specific blood tests: ESR increased markedly in temporal arteritis and is the first-line investigation
			• Other blood tests: FBC, CRP
			• Biopsy: of temporal artery if indicated. Shows giant cell infiltration
				• Prednisolone for temporal arteritis

Continued overleaf

Table 5.1 Sudden painless visual loss

TABLE 5.1. **Sudden painless visual loss** (*continued*).

Disease	Cause	Features	Investigations	Treatment
Retinal detachment	• Trauma – particularly acceleration–deceleration injuries • Retinal tears • Positive family history • Complication of cataract surgery • Myopia (high level)	• There are three different ways in which retinal detachment may manifest. Remember as **RET**inal: **R** – **R**hegmatogenous **E** – **E**xudative **T** – **T**ractional • Symptoms may be remembered as the **4Fs**: **F** – **F**loaters **F** – **F**lashes (photopsia) **F** – **F**ield loss **F** – **F**all in acuity occurs when macula detaches • Superior temporal quadrant most commonly affected	• Visual acuity • Pupil analysis: may demonstrate a relative afferent pupillary defect or a Marcus Gunn pupil if not consensual • Visual field analysis • Anterior slit lamp examination • Fundoscopy: visualizes detached portion of the retina (grey opalescent)	Emergency care **Surgical:** • Reattach the retina (e.g. vitrectomy with gas tamponade)

Table 5.1. Sudden painless visual loss

| Occlusion of the retinal artery | • Temporal arteritis
• Atherosclerosis
• Risk factors increase with atrial fibrillation, coagulopathies and sickle cell disease | • Sudden painless central visual loss | • Perform blood tests to detect the underlying cause (e.g. FBC, sickle cell studies, ESR, CRP, prothrombin time, activated partial thromboplastin time, cholesterol and triglyceride levels)
• ECG: for atrial fibrillation
• Full ophthalmology assessment as above | Treatment depends on the time elapsed since visual loss detected. Retinal artery occlusion requires prompt emergency treatment:
• Lower IOP: ocular massage, anterior chamber paracentesis
• Other medications: timolol, acetazolamide, mannitol, thrombolytics may be useful, hyperbaric oxygen therapy (within 2–12 hours of onset) |
| Vitreous haemorrhage | • Diabetes mellitus
• Coagulation disorders | • Sudden painless visual loss: 'cobwebs and floaters'
• Photophobia
• Photopsia | | Treat underlying cause

Conservative:
• Bed rest with the head of the bed elevated 30–45°

Medical:
• Depends on underlying cause

Surgical:
• Laser therapy
• Cryotherapy
• Vitrectomy |

Table 5.1: Sudden painless visual loss

MAP 5.1. Macular degeneration

What is macular degeneration?
This is a chronic ocular condition, which is more common in older patients. There are three different types:

1. Dry (geographic) macular degeneration:
   - Characteristic yellow drusen.
   - Most common type.

2. Wet (exudative) macular degeneration:
   - Severe and accelerative.
   - Associated with neovascularization of the choroid and, therefore, haemorrhage.

3. Stargardt macular degeneration:
   - Occurs in teenagers.
   - Rare.

Causes
Unknown. There are theories which suggest that VEGF plays a role in the pathophysiology of the disease and there is a link with smoking (increases the risk by 3.6).

MAP 5.1. **Macular degeneration**

Symptoms
- Progressive central visual loss.
- Scotomas.
- Visual acuity: decreased.
- Metamorphopsia.

Investigations
- Ophthalmology examination:
  ○ Visual acuity.
  ○ Visual fields.
  ○ Amsler grid: metamorphopsia.
  ○ Fluorescein angiography: wet macular degeneration (neovascularization).
- Blood tests: FBC, U&E, glucose, cholesterol and lipid levels.

Risk factors: remember as **ABCS:**

A – **A**ge: generally over 60
B – high **B**lood pressure
C – increased **C**holesterol levels/
    Caucasian ethnicity
S – **S**moking/**S**unlight (UV) exposure

Complications
- Blindness.
- Depression.

Treatment

Treatment	Dry	Wet
Conservative	Patient education Referral to occupational therapy to improve quality of life (e.g. adapted house aids such as magnified home appliances)	As with dry macular degeneration
Medical	No effective treatment	Oral vitamins and antioxidants Anti-VEGF therapy (e.g. ranibizumab)
Surgical	No effective treatment	Photodynamic therapy

MAP 5.1. Macular degeneration

MAP 5.2. Glaucoma

What is glaucoma?

Glaucoma comprises a group of ocular disorders characterized by the following triad:

- Visual field loss (nasal and superior fields affected first).
- Optic disc cupping.
- Optic nerve damage.

IOP is often raised but it may be normal.

Causes

There are two types of glaucoma: open angle (most common) and closed angle. The following table explores the differences between the two.

Feature	Open angle	Closed angle
Cause	Primary: • *MYOC* mutation Secondary: • Trauma – obstruction to the trabecular meshwork	Primary: • Shallow anterior chambers Secondary: • Trauma • Tumour of the ciliary body
Pathology	Drainage of aqueous humour through the trabecular meshwork is restricted	Outflow of aqueous humour is obstructed since iris bows against the trabecular meshwork
Painful	No	Yes
Associations	Myopia	Hypermetropia

Symptoms

- Glaucoma may be picked up on routine ophthalmology examination.
- Diminished vision.
- Closed angle glaucoma: hazy cornea, semidilated pupil.
- Pain.
- Key triad: 1, visual field loss; 2, alteration to the optic nerve cup; and 3, alteration to the optic disc.

Investigations

- Tonometry: measures IOP.
- Fundoscopy.
- Visual field assessment.
- Cup-to-disc ratio.
- Gonioscopy: assesses the iridocorneal angle.
- Scanning laser ophthalmoscopy.
- Scanning laser polarimetry.

Complication
- Blindness.

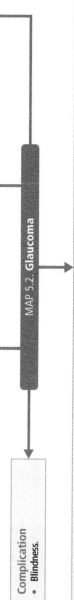

MAP 5.2. Glaucoma

Treatment

Conservative: patient education and annual assessment

Medical:

Class	Example	MOA	Side effects
Beta blockers	Betaxolol	↓ IOP by slowing the rate of aqueous humour production	Contraindicated in asthma, heart block and bradycardia
Prostaglandin analogues	Latanoprost	↓ IOP by increasing uveoscleral outflow	Brown pigmentation of iris, ↓ visual acuity
Sympathomimetics	Brimonidine	Selective α_2-adrenoreceptor agonist; ↓ IOP by slowing the rate of aqueous humour production and by increasing uveoscleral outflow	↓ visual acuity, itching, diplopia, redness of the eyelid, excessive tearing, tunnel vision
Carbonic anhydrase inhibitors	Acetazolamide	Inhibits carbonic anhydrase, therefore ↓ IOP by slowing the rate of aqueous humour production	Weak systemic diuretic. Is a sulphonamide derivative, therefore sulphonamide side effects (e.g. rashes)
Miotics	Pilocarpine	↓ IOP by opening drainage channels in trabecular meshwork	Blurred vision, ciliary spasm, itching and lens changes (with chronic use)

MAP 5.2. Glaucoma

MAP 5.3.   Cataracts

What are cataracts?

A cataract is opacity of the crystalline lens and is a leading worldwide cause of blindness. There are many different types of cataracts and these may be defined based on location or causative disease. Some examples are provided below.

Location:

- Nuclear cataract.
- Subcapsular cataract.
- Cortical cataract.

Associated with disease:

- Diabetes: snowflake cataract.
- Wilson's disease: sunflower cataract.

Causes

There are many different causes and risk factors for the development of cataracts. These may be congenital or acquired.

Congenital:

- TORCHES infections (see Map 2.6, p. 50).
- Genetic causes:
  o Trisomies.
  o Galactosaemia.
  o Lowe's syndrome.

Symptoms

- Leukocoria.
- Decreased visual acuity.
- Diplopia.
- Glare.
- Myopic shift.
- Nystagmus (congenital cataracts).

Investigations

- Ophthalmic examination.
- Blood tests: to uncover the underlying cause; FBC, U&E, LFTs, glucose, cholesterol levels +/– specific tests (e.g. copper studies for Wilson's disease or urine amino acids, phosphate and calcium for Lowe's syndrome).

MAP 5.3.   **Cataracts**

Acquired: remember VITAMIN D:

V – Vascular complications (e.g. hypertension).

I – Infection (e.g. onchocerciasis [river blindness]).

T – Trauma (e.g. UV exposure, blunt force).

A – Autoimmune (e.g. hypoparathyroidism), Age

M – Metabolic (e.g. diabetes mellitus, Wilson's disease).

I – Irradiation

N – Never forget drugs (e.g. side effect of corticosteroids)

D – Dermatology (e.g. eczema).

Treatment

Conservative:
- Patient education and annual ophthalmic review.

Medical:
- Treatment of underlying cause (e.g. penicillamine for Wilson's disease).

Surgical:
- Phacoemulsification may only be performed on ripe cataracts and then an intraocular lens is implanted.

Complications
- Blindness.
- Complications of cataract surgery (e.g. retinal detachment).

TABLE 5.2. **Red eye.** There are many causes of red eye. These are outlined below.

Disease	Cause	Features	Investigations	Treatment
Acute angle closure glaucoma	See Map 5.2 (p. 164)	See Map 5.2 (p. 164)	See Map 5.2 (p. 164)	See Map 5.2 (p. 164)
Anterior uveitis	Associated with HLA-B27 Some examples include: **ABCS:** A – **A**nkylosing spondylitis, juvenile idiopathic **A**rthritis, psoriatic **A**rthritis, reactive **A**rthritis B – **B**ehçet's disease C – **C**rohn's disease S – **S**arcoidosis, **S**ystemic lupus erythematosus	• Painful red eye • Acute onset • Photophobia • Blurred vision • Fixed oval pupil	Investigations to establish underlying cause Fundoscopy Radiology: x-ray may be useful in cases of arthritis	**Conservative:** • Patient education **Medical:** • Treatment of underlying cause • Specific treatment of anterior uveitis: corticosteroids and cycloplegics may be used
Scleritis	Associated with autoimmune diseases such as rheumatoid arthritis and Sjögren's syndrome	• Painful red eye • Pain worse on movement • Diminished visual acuity	Investigations to establish underlying cause Full ophthalmic examination Differentiate scleritis from episcleritis by administering phenylephrine eye drops. In episcleritis blood vessels turn pale	**Conservative:** • Patient education **Medical:** • Treatment of underlying cause • Specific treatment of scleritis: NSAIDs, corticosteroids

Table 5.2. Red eye

		Clinical diagnosis	**Conservative:**
Conjunctivitis	**Bacterial:** • *Staphylococcus* spp. • *Streptococcus* spp. • *Chlamydia trachomatis* **Viral:** • Influenza • HSV • VZV **Allergic** **Autoimmune:** • Associated with conditions such as reactive arthritis **Occupational exposure:** • Exposure to chemicals	• Itchy, red eye • Bacterial: purulent, sticky discharge • Viral: clear discharge	• Patient education **Medical:** • Bacterial: antibiotic eye drops • Viral: self-limiting • Allergic: antihistamines • Autoimmune: artificial tears and treatment of underlying cause • Occupational exposure: irrigation of chemical with saline solution
Subconjunctival haemorrhage	Remember as **ABCDE:** A – **A**cute haemorrhagic conjunctivitis B – increased **B**lood pressure C – **C**oughing D – **D**isorders of coagulation E – **E**ye trauma	• Red eye	Clinical diagnosis	**Conservative:** • Patient education • Advise that it looks more alarming than it is **Medical:** • Self-limiting condition • Artificial tears may sometimes be given

Table 5.2 Red eye

Table 5.3. Diabetic eye disease

TABLE 5.3. **Diabetic eye disease. This is a microvascular complication of diabetes mellitus.**

Pathophysiology: hyperglycaemia ⇒ vascular pericyte loss and endothelial damage ⇒ microaneurysm formation ⇒ retinal ischaemia ⇒ stimulation of growth factors ⇒ neovascularization.

The features that are characteristic of each phase of diabetic retinopathy are explored below.

Phase	Feature
Background	Remember as **ABCDE:** A – micro**A**neuryms (dots) B – **B**lot haemorrhages <3 C – **C**otton wool spots (oedema from retinal infarcts) D – venous **D**ilatation E – hard **E**xudates
Pre-proliferative	Remember as **ABCD:** A – micro**A**neuyms (dots). More than background retinopathy B – venous **B**eading and looping C – **C**otton wool spots >5 D – **D**ark cluster haemorrhages
Proliferative	Neovascularization Fibrous proliferation Haemorrhages
Advanced	Retinal detachment Rubeosis iridis Neovascular glaucoma
Maculopathy	As above but involves the macular

MAP 6.1a. Hearing loss (flow chart)

MAP 6.1a. **Hearing loss (flow chart)**

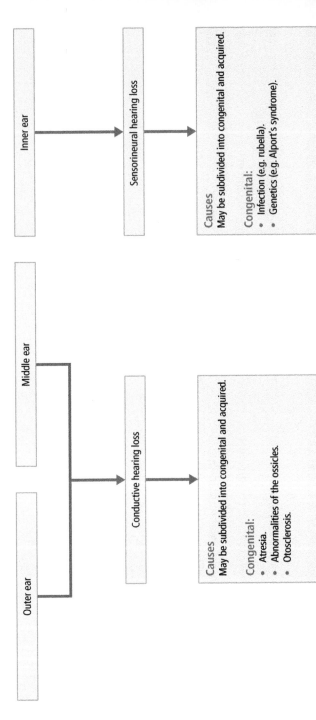

Outer ear

Middle ear

Inner ear

Conductive hearing loss

Sensorineural hearing loss

Causes
May be subdivided into congenital and acquired.

Congenital:
- Atresia.
- Abnormalities of the ossicles.
- Otosclerosis.

Causes
May be subdivided into congenital and acquired.

Congenital:
- Infection (e.g. rubella).
- Genetics (e.g. Alport's syndrome).

Acquired

- Wax.
- Otitis externa.
- Glue ear (see Map 6.2, p. 176).
- Perforated drum.

Acquired

- Presbycusis.
- Infection (e.g. meningitis, measles).
- Trauma (e.g. noise injury, head trauma).
- Tumour (e.g. acoustic neuroma).
- Ototoxic drugs (e.g. gentamicin, furosemide, cisplatin).
- Ménière's disease (see Map 6.1b, p. 174).

MAP 6.1a. Hearing loss (flow chart)

Glue ear

What is glue ear?
Glue ear, also known as otitis media with effusion, is a collection of fluid within the middle ear. This fluid is thought to occur due to dysfunctional Eustachian tubes, which create negative pressure. It occurs in males more than females.

Cause
The exact cause is unknown. It often occurs secondary to a viral upper respiratory tract infection or acute bacterial otitis media.

Risk factors: remember as EARS:
E – Eustachian tube abnormalities
(e.g. in Down's syndrome)
A – Adenoids (enlarged)
R – Respiratory infections
S – Smoking (usually parents), Season (winter)

Symptoms
May vary depending on age of child/adult. Bulging drum of varying colour. A fluid level may be present.

Ménière's disease

What is Ménière's disease?
Ménière's disease, also known as endolymphatic hydrops, is a cause of sensorineural hearing loss. It is thought to be caused by the dilatation and excessive fluid collection within the endolymphatic spaces. It is more common in females than males and presents more commonly in middle aged adults.

Cause.
The exact cause is unknown.

Symptoms.
Presents with a characteristic triad:
1. Vertigo.
2. Low pitch tinnitus.
3. Sensorineural hearing loss.
Other features include aural fullness, a positive Romberg test and nystagmus.

Investigations.
Clinical diagnosis but also perform MRI of head to rule out space-occupying lesion.

Treatment
Conservative: patient education.

Medical: acute attacks – cyclizine or prochlorperazine; long-term treatment – betahistine or thiazide drugs; treat symptoms (e.g. vomiting with prochlorperazine).

Surgical: endolymphatic shunts; ototoxic drugs.

MAP 6.1b. **Hearing loss (specific conditions)**

Otosclerosis

What is otosclerosis? This is an autosomal dominant condition that typically affects females aged 20–40 years.

Causes. Hereditary. Normal ossicle bone is replaced by vascular bone, which is spongy.

Symptoms. Conductive hearing loss, tinnitus, flamingo tinge appearance to the tympanic membrane (Schwart's sign).

Investigation. Audiometry.

Treatment:
* Conservative: patient education.
* Medical: sodium fluoride.
* Surgical: stapedectomy.

Investigations

Audiograms (conductive defects), impedance audiometry.

Treatment

Conservative:
* Often self-limiting.
* Hearing aids only if bilateral symptoms.

Medical:
* NICE does not recommend antibiotics.

Surgical:
* Myringotomy.
* Grommets +/– adenoidectomy.

MAP 6.1b. Hearing loss (specific conditions)

MAP 6.2. Benign paroxysmal positional vertigo (BPPV)

What is benign paroxysmal positional vertigo?
This pathology of the inner ear results in the sudden onset of nausea, vertigo and nystagmus following certain movements of the head.

Causes
BPPV is thought to be caused by the displacement of otoconia (small calcium carbonate crystals) from the utricle into the semicircular canals. Movement of these crystals along the canal in question stimulates the sensation of rotation.

Risk factors
There are many factors that contribute to the displacement of otoconia. The commonest is head injury, but others include infection and degeneration attributed to old age.

Symptoms
- Vertigo.
- Nausea.
- Lightheadedness.
- Imbalance.
- Nystagmus.

The above symptoms are nearly always precipitated by a sudden change in head position, such as lying down.

Investigations
A diagnosis is made depending on symptoms, patient history and examination.

- Dix–Hallpike test – a positive test stimulates bursts of nystagmus.
- Undertake vestibular and auditory tests.

MAP 6.2. Benign paroxysmal positional vertigo (BPPV)

Treatment

Conservative:
- Patient education – said to be a self-limiting condition that may resolve in ~2 months after onset.
- Epley manoeuvre – attempts to reposition the displaced otoconia.

Medical:
- Anti-emetics for nausea if severe.

Surgical:
- Very rarely performed and should not be considered unless the above methods have failed. Examples include posterior canal plugging.

Complication
- Dizziness, therefore increased risk of falls.

MAP 6.2 Benign paroxysmal positional vertigo (BPPV)

What is epistaxis?

Epistaxis is the term used for nosebleed. It is very common and there are two major types:

1. Anterior epistaxis: most common. Often presents as unilateral nasal bleeding and occurs from Kiesselbach's plexus (also known as Little's area).
2. Posterior epistaxis: less common but more difficult to manage. Presents with bilateral nasal bleeding and also post-nasal bleeding into the oropharynx.

Causes

There are many different causes of nosebleeds ranging from the idiopathic to foreign bodies and tumours. Some causes are listed below.
Remember as **EPISTAXIS:**

E – Epistaxis past history (e.g. anatomical deformities or hereditary haemorrhagic telangiectasia)

P – Punch to the face/trauma

I – Inflammatory reactions (e.g. recent upper respiratory tract infection)

S – Systemic factors (e.g. hypertension)

T – Thrombocytopenia

A – Alcohol – causes vasodilation

X – factor X deficiency

I – Intranasal tumours

S – Sprays (e.g. prolonged use of nasal steroids)

Symptoms

- Haemorrhage of varying severity from one or both nostrils.
- Presence of blood in the oropharynx.

Treatment

Conservative:

- ABCDE – emergency care.
- Pinch fleshy parts of the nose together and tilt head forward. Place an ice pack on the bridge of the nose or the back of the neck. Do this for 20–30 minutes.

Medical:

- Anterior epistaxis:
  - Adrenaline solution to clean the nose and cause vasoconstriction. Reassess to identify bleed.
  - Silver nitrate sticks – used for nasal cautery if bleeding point clearly identified. Apply to this point and a small area around it. **Caution:** do not use bilaterally since there is a risk of nasal perforation. Always prescribe Naseptin cream after cautery. This consists of neomycin and chloramphenicol. Contraindications: peanut allergy.
  - If bleeding still perfuse after cautery, then consider nasal packing with either (1) Rapid Rhino®, (2) Merocel® or (3) BIPP gauze.

MAP 6.3. Epistaxis

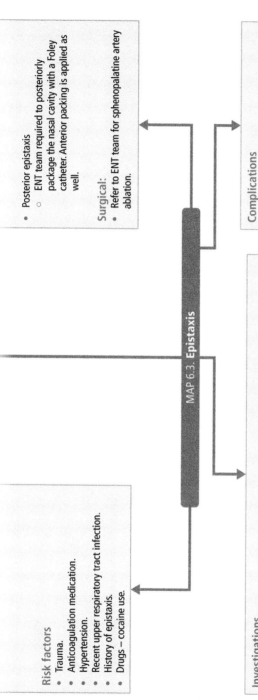

MAP 6.3. Epistaxis

Risk factors
- Trauma.
- Anticoagulation medication.
- Hypertension.
- Recent upper respiratory tract infection.
- History of epistaxis.
- Drugs – cocaine use.

Investigations

It is essential in all cases to examine both nostrils with a nasal speculum and a pen torch to identify whether bleeding is unilateral or bilateral, as well as identifying the source of the bleed. It is also vital to assess whether post-nasal bleeding has compromised breathing.

In most acute cases specific tests are unnecessary. However, recurrent cases require:

- Blood tests: FBC, coagulation studies.
- Radiology: CT (if malignancy suspected).
- Other: nasopharyngoscopy (if malignancy suspected).

- Posterior epistaxis
  ○ ENT team required to posteriorly package the nasal cavity with a Foley catheter. Anterior packing is applied as well.

Surgical:
- Refer to ENT team for sphenopalatine artery ablation.

Complications
- Compromise to airway.
- Anaemia.

MAP 6.4. Nasopharyngeal cancer

What is nasopharyngeal cancer?

Nasopharyneal cancer is typically a squamous cell carcinoma (85%). Other cell types include adenocarcinoma, lymphoma and melanoma.
It is more common in Asian populations and in males.

Causes

The exact cause of nasopharyngeal tumours is unknown but risk factors include:
- Genetics: HLA-A2.
- Infection: Epstein–Barr virus.
- Diet: nitrosamines and vitamin C deficiency.

Symptoms

Remember as **NOSE:**

N – **N**eck lump

O – Otalgia, nasal **O**bstruction

S – **S**ymptoms of spread (e.g. nerve palsies – mandibular nerve; cranial nerves – most commonly CNs V, VI and XII; Horner's syndrome).

E – **E**pistaxis.

MAP 6.4. **Nasopharyngeal cancer**

Investigations

- Blood tests: FBC, WCC, U&E, LFTs, ESR, Epstein–Barr virus and viral capsid antigen.
- Specific tests: audiogram, tympanogram and visual fields.
- Radiology: CT, MRI with TNM classification. Angiography for angiofibroma.

Complications

- Metastasis.
- Invasion of local structures.
- Death.

Treatment

Conservative:
- Patient education, Macmillan nurses referral.

Medical:
- Chemotherapy and radiotherapy.

Surgical:
- For angiofibroma.

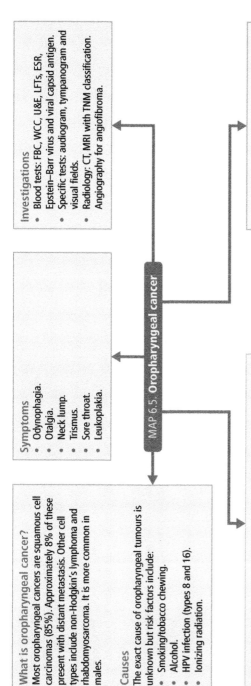

What is oropharyngeal cancer?

Most oropharyngeal cancers are squamous cell carcinomas (85%). Approximately 8% of these present with distant metastasis. Other cell types include non-Hodgkin's lymphoma and rhabdomyosarcoma. It is more common in males.

Causes

The exact cause of oropharyngeal tumours is unknown but risk factors include:
- Smoking/tobacco chewing.
- Alcohol.
- HPV infection (types 8 and 16).
- Ionizing radiation.

Symptoms
- Odynophagia.
- Otalgia.
- Neck lump.
- Trismus.
- Sore throat.
- Leukoplakia.

MAP 6.5. Oropharyngeal cancer

Investigations
- Blood tests: FBC, WCC, U&E, LFTs, ESR, Epstein–Barr virus and viral capsid antigen.
- Specific tests: audiogram, tympanogram and visual fields.
- Radiology: CT, MRI with TNM classification. Angiography for angiofibroma.

Complications
- Metastasis.
- Invasion of local structures.
- Death.

Treatment

Treatment depends on the cell type and the TNM grading.
- Squamous cell carcinoma: radiotherapy and surgery.
- Carcinoma of the soft palate: T1/T2 – radiotherapy; T3/4 – resection.
- Posterior pharyngeal wall carcinoma: T1/2 – radical radiotherapy, resection.
- Tonsil carcinoma: T1/2 – radical radiotherapy, transoral surgery; T3/4 – resection +/– dissection and reconstruction.
- Postoperative radiotherapy required for nodal involvement.

MAP 6.5. Oropharyngeal cancer

MAP 6.6. Laryngeal cancer

What is laryngeal cancer?

Laryngeal tumours may be benign or malignant:

- Malignant: squamous cell carcinoma, adenocarcinoma, sarcoma, verrucous carcinoma, undifferentiated.
- Benign: papillomas, chondromas, lipomas.

Causes

The exact cause of laryngeal tumours is unknown but risk factors include:

- Age.
- Male.
- Smoking.
- Alcohol.

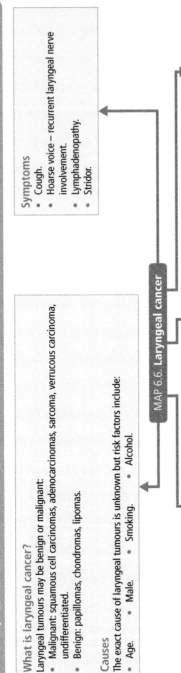

MAP 6.6. **Laryngeal cancer**

Symptoms

- Cough.
- Hoarse voice – recurrent laryngeal nerve involvement.
- Lymphadenopathy.
- Stridor.

Complications

- Metastasis.
- Invasion of local structures.
- Death.
- Vocal cord paralysis.

Investigations

- Blood tests: FBC, WCC, U&E, LFTs, ESR.
- Specific tests: examination under anaesthesia and biopsy.
- Radiology: chest x-ray, CT, MRI.

Treatment

Conservative:

- Patient education, Macmillan nurses referral.
- Speech therapy after chemotherapy, radiotherapy and surgery.

Medical:

- Treatment of laryngeal cancer is dictated by the TMN stage.
- Radiotherapy and chemotherapy.

Surgical:

- Larynx sparing surgery (e.g. endoscopic laser resection, laryngofissure, cordectomy, vertical partial laryngectomy).
- Total or partial laryngectomy.
- Neck dissection.

Map 7.1. Atopic eczema

What is atopic eczema?

Eczema is a common chronic inflammatory skin condition that presents with itchy, dry, scaly lesions. Atopic eczema is the most common type of eczema, but there are other variations, such as contact dermatitis, as well as those that are defined by appearance such as discoid eczema and venous eczema.

Causes

The exact cause of atopic eczema is not known. It is thought to be multifactorial and is generally considered to be an interaction between genetic components and the immune system.

- **Genetic:** increased risk with a positive family history. Filaggrin gene mutations predispose to eczema.
- **Allergen exposure:** e.g. certain washing detergents, perfumes, food allergies.
- **Exacerbating factors:** emotional stress, temperature fluctuation.

Symptoms

- Xerosis (generalized dry skin).
- Erythematous lesions.
- Excoriation.
- Lichenifications.
- Signs of superadded infection (e.g. vesicles).
- Itching.
- Note distribution:
  - Face – often in babies.
  - Antecubital fossa.
  - Popliteal fossa.
  - Wrists.
  - Ankles.
- Nails – polished from scratching.

Investigations

- Always ask about other atopic conditions such as asthma and hay fever as well as food allergy.
- Blood tests: serum IgE (high).
- Other: skin prick or RAST.
- Swab – to identify causative organism if infection present.

MAP 7.1. **Atopic eczema**

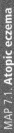

Treatment

Conservative:

- Patient education and avoidance of triggering factors.

Medical:

- Emollients – wet wraps may be used to aid absorption.
- Topical steroids – use lowest potency first.
- Antibiotics – for secondary bacterial infection.
- Anti-virals – aciclovir is used in eczema herpeticum.
- PUVA treatment may be used in resistant cases.

Complications

- Chronic dry skin.
- Superadded infection:
  - Usually *Staphylococcus aureus* resulting in impetiginized eczema.
  - Herpes simplex virus may cause eczema herpeticum.
- Eye problems such as conjunctivitis and blepharitis.
- Decreased quality of sleep.

Map 7.1. Atopic eczema

Map 7.2 Seborrhoeic dermatitis

What is seborrhoeic dermatitis?
This is a chronic inflammatory skin condition resulting in dermatitis in areas rich in sebaceous glands, such as the nasolabial folds.

Causes
The exact cause of seborrhoeic dermatitis is not known but current theories suggest that the yeast *Malassezia furfur* plays a role. Additionally, seborrhoeic dermatitis is more common in patients suffering with HIV and, therefore, a weakened immune system may play a role.

Symptoms
- Red/white/yellow, scaly lesions present usually around the nasolabial folds, eyebrows, chest and scalp. May also occur in other hair bearing areas and in flexural folds.
- Itching.
- Cradle cap – seen in babies.

Investigations
Seborrhoeic dermatitis tends to be a clinical diagnosis.
- Skin scraping microscopy – may show *Malassezia furfur*.
- Skin swabs for superadded infection, usually *Staphylococcus aureus*.

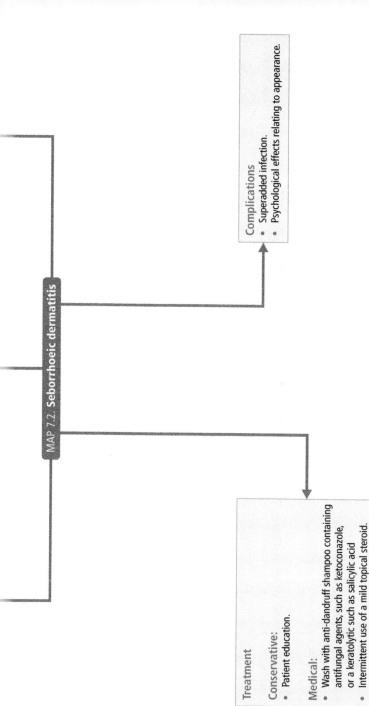

MAP 7.2. **Seborrhoeic dermatitis**

Complications
- Superadded infection.
- Psychological effects relating to appearance.

Treatment

Conservative:
- Patient education.

Medical:
- Wash with anti-dandruff shampoo containing antifungal agents, such as ketoconazole, or a keratolytic such as salicylic acid
- Intermittent use of a mild topical steroid.

Map 7.2. Seborrhoeic dermatitis

Map 7.3. Psoriasis

What is psoriasis?

Psoriasis is a chronic, non-infectious inflammatory skin condition characterized by well-demarcated salmon pink plaques with silvery scales. It is very common and may occur at any age. Two peaks have been identified – in the 20s and 50s. Males and females are equally affected. This condition causes hyperproliferation of the epidermis, inflammation of the epidermis and dermis as well as retention of nuclei in keratinocytes in the horny layer (parakeratosis).

Causes

The exact cause of psoriasis is unknown but broadly it is thought to be due to a complex interaction between genetics and environmental triggers.

- Genetic factors:
  - Mutations of *PSORS1* on chromosome 6 – associated more with guttate psoriasis.
  - Polymorphisms in genes for IL-12 and IL-23.

Symptoms

- General symptoms: itching, pain, decreased dexterity.
- Lesion type:
  1. Chronic plaque psoriasis – extensor surfaces.
     - Psoriasis gyrate – curved linear patterns.
     - Annular psoriasis – ring-like lesions, central clearing.
     - Psoriasis follicularis – scaly papules at pilosebaceous follicles.
  2. Rupioid plaques – limpet shell appearance, 2–5 cm.
  3. Ostraceous psoriasis – oyster shell appearance.
  4. Inverse psoriasis – intertriginous areas.
  5. Guttate psoriasis – raindrop appearance over body. Associated with prior streptococcal pharyngitis. Usually younger patients.
  6. Pustular psoriasis – palms and soles usually.
  7. Erythrodermic psoriasis – dermatological emergency.

Treatment

Conservative:

- Patient education. Avoid triggering factors (e.g. smoking is strongly linked with palmoplantar psoriasis)
- Provide information on treatment options and monitor bloods regularly, especially when patients are taking systemic therapy or biological agents. Also, be aware of teratogenicity in women of child-bearing age.
- Assess severity:
  - Patient's perspective: assessed using the Dermatology Life Quality Index (DLQI).
  - Physician's perspective: assessed using the Psoriasis Area and Severity Index (PASI).

Medical:

- Topical therapy: emollients, keratolytic agents, Goeckerman treatment (coal tar and UVB), dithranol treatment (short contact therapy), topical steroids (e.g. betamethasone ointment, calcipotriol with and without betamethasone).

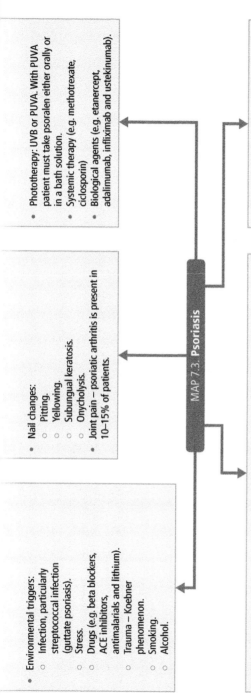

MAP 7.3. Psoriasis

- Environmental triggers:
  - Infection, particularly streptococcal infection (guttate psoriasis).
  - Stress.
  - Drugs (e.g. beta blockers, ACE inhibitors, antimalarials and lithium).
  - Trauma – Koebner phenomenon.
  - Smoking.
  - Alcohol.

- Nail changes:
  - Pitting.
  - Yellowing.
  - Subungual keratosis.
  - Onycholysis.
- Joint pain – psoriatic arthritis is present in 10–15% of patients.

- Phototherapy: UVB or PUVA. With PUVA patient must take psoralen either orally or in a bath solution.
- Systemic therapy (e.g. methotrexate, ciclosporin)
- Biological agents (e.g. etanercept, adalimumab, infliximab and ustekinumab).

Complications
- Psoriatic arthritis.
- Eye disease (e.g. blepharitis and conjunctivitis).
- Increased risk of:
  - Cardiovascular disease.
  - Metabolic syndrome.
  - Depression.

Investigations
Diagnosis is usually based on clinical examination.
- Well-demarcated salmon pink plaques with silvery white scales.
- Usually over extensor surfaces but also may be present on the scalp and navel.
- White blanching ring present on skin surrounding plaque. This is called Woronoff's ring.
- Nail changes: (see symptoms).
- Special signs:
  - Auspitz's sign: capillary bleeding when individual scales removed from plaque.
  - Koebner's phenomenon: new lesions at site of trauma.
  - Bulkeley's membrane: moist red surface on removal of scales.

MAP 7.4. Pityriasis

Pityriasis versicolor

What is pityriasis versicolor?

This is a commensal yeast infection of the skin that causes numerous lesions of varying colours on the trunk and back.

Causes

The yeasts *Malassezia globosa* and *Malassezia furfur*. Triggering factors include excessive sweating and living in hot climates as well as immunosuppression.

Symptoms
- Mild itching.
- Bran-like scales of varying colour.

Pityriasis rosea

What is pityriasis rosea?

This is a benign, self-limiting bran-like scaly rash that occurs on the trunk.

Causes

The exact cause of this condition is unknown, but HHV-7 has been implicated.

Symptoms
- Itching.
- 70% of patients have an upper respiratory tract infection before dermatological symptoms present.
- Herald patch – a single, larger lesion precedes smaller oval plaques. It is pink in appearance and has a central clearing.
- Smaller oval lesions follow a 'Christmas tree' distribution.

Investigations
Usually a clinical diagnosis.

Treatment
Often no treatment is required since it is a self-limiting condition.

Conservative:
- Patient education that condition is benign.

Medical:
- Anti-histamines or steroid to aid itching.

Investigations
Usually a clinical diagnosis.
- Fungal cultures for *Malassezia*.
- Wood lamp examination – yellow-green fluorescence in affected regions.

Treatment

Conservative:
- Patient education.

Medical:
- Topical anti-fungal agents/shampoos.
- Propylene glycol solution.
- Sodium thiosulphate solution.
- Oral anti-fungal agents in extensive disease.

Map 7.4. Pityriasis

Map 7.5. Erythematous lesions

MAP 7.5. **Erythematous lesions**

Erythema multiforme

What is erythema multiforme?

This is a skin condition that is caused by a hypersensitivity reaction. There are varying degrees of severity:

1. Erythema multiforme minor – least severe.
2. Erythema multiforme major.
3. Stevens–Johnson syndrome (SJS) <10% body surface area; toxic epidermal necrolysis (TEN) >30% body surface area – potentially life-threatening.

Causes

The exact cause remains unknown in 50% of cases. Some specific causes include:

- Bacterial infections (e.g. *Streptococcus*, *Neisseria meningitidis*).
- Viral infections (e.g. herpes simplex virus).
- Fungal (e.g. *Coccidiodes immitis*).
- Parasitic infection (e.g. *Toxoplasma gondii*).
- Adverse drug reactions (e.g. penicillin, sulphonamides, aspirin, allopurinol).
- Malignancies – non-Hodgkin's lymphoma, multiple myeloma, leukaemia.

Symptoms

- Multiple erythematous plaques appearing as concentric rings in a symmetrical distribution.
- SJS: fever >39°C; fatigue; lesions in the mucous membranes; conjunctivitis.

Erythema nodosum

What is erythema nodosum?

This is an immune-mediated disorder resulting in a panniculitis.

Causes

There are many varying causes of erythema nodosum. Remember as NODOSUM:

N – No cause found
O – Occult malignancy
D – Drugs (e.g. sulphonamides, oral contraceptive pill)
O – Other infections (e.g. streptococcal pharyngitis)
S – Sarcoidosis
U – Ulcerative colitis/Crohn's disease
M – *Mycobacterium*

Symptoms

Painful red nodules on the anterior surface of the shin.

Investigations

Identify the underlying cause.

- Throat swab.
- Acid fast bacillus staining (Ziehl–Nielsen) if TB suspected.
- Blood tests – FBC, WCC, U&E, LFTs, CRP, ASO titres, viral studies.
- Radiology – chest x-ray.

Investigations

Not essential to make the diagnosis, but vital for monitoring, especially in SJS.

- Blood tests – FBC (↓), WCC (↓), eosinophils (↑), LFTs (↑), viral titres.
- Urinalysis – mild proteinuria.

Treatment

Conservative:

- Remove causative agent.
- Use the SCORTEN score to predict mortality in SJS and TEN.
- Incise and drain large bullae.

Medical:

- Erythema multiforme minor – topical steroids and oral antihistamines
- Erythema multiforme major – intravenous fluids, mouthwash (antiseptic and analgesic).
- SJS – intravenous fluids, mouthwash (antiseptic and analgesic), ophthalmology review, genital care with catheterization, assessment and treatment of superadded infection.

Complications

- Dehydration and electrolyte imbalance.
- Acute respiratory distress syndrome.
- Eye problems (e.g. conjunctivitis, corneal ulcers, symblepharon).
- Renal failure.

Treatment

Conservative:

- Compression stockings.

Medical:

- Treatment of underlying cause.
- Analgesia.

Complications

Serious complications are rare.

Map 7.5. Erythematous lesions

Map 7.6. Lichenoid lesions

MAP 7.6. Lichenoid lesions

Lichen planus

What is lichen planus?

Lichen planus is a chronic inflammatory skin condition characterized by well-demarcated purple papules present on mucous membranes, flexor surfaces and the genital area. It has a symmetrical distribution.

There are many clinical classifications of lichen planus including, but not limited to, cutaneous lichen planus, mucosal lichen planus, lichen planopilaris and lichen planus of the nails.

Causes

Lichen planus is thought to be a T-cell mediated autoimmune disease. Research has suggested some contributing factors such as:

- Genetic predisposition – HLA-DR1.
- Trauma.
- Viral infection – HSV, hepatitis C.

Symptoms

- Polygonal purple papules in specific regions such as the wrists, shins, lower back and genital region.
- Oral mucosal involvement – Wickham's striae.
- Scarring alopecia.
- Nail lesions – onycholysis, thinning, ridging, pterygium, anonychia.

Lichen sclerosus

What is lichen sclerosus?

It is a chronic skin condition that results in thinning of the epithelium, particularly in the genital region of women.

Causes

The exact cause of lichen sclerosus is unknown but several risk factors have been proposed such as:

- Genetic predisposition.
- Previous history of autoimmune conditions (e.g. thyroid disease, type 1 diabetes mellitus, vitiligo).
- Low oestrogen status – due to higher prevalence in post-menopausal women.

Symptoms

- Anogenital lesions – atrophic white macules.
- Fissures.
- Excoriations.

Investigations

Typically a clinical diagnosis. A biopsy may be needed to confirm diagnosis and assess for cancer.

Investigations

Typically a clinical diagnosis. A biopsy may be needed to confirm diagnosis and assess for cancer.

Treatment

Conservative:
- Patient education.
- Drug cessation if responsible for lichen planus-like reaction (e.g. antibiotics [tetracycline], anti-rheumatic drugs [penicillamine]).

Medical:
- Topic treatments – steroids, calcineurin inhibitors, tacrolimus ointment, retinoids.
- Systemic – oral prednisolone, methotrexate, azathioprine.

Complications
- Increased risk of squamous cell carcinoma.

Treatment

Conservative:
- Patient education – wash regularly, wear loose clothing.
- Photographic monitoring of lesion.

Medical:
- Topic treatments – emollients, steroids, calcineurin inhibitors, tacrolimus ointment, retinoids.
- Systemic – oral prednisolone, retinoids, methotrexate, ciclosporin.

Complications
- Increased risk of squamous cell carcinoma.
- Adhesions and scarring:
  - Phimosis.
  - Introital stenosis.
  - Labia minora shrinkage.

Map 7.6. Lichenoid lesions

MAP 7.7. Bullous disorders

Bullous pemphigus

What is bullous pemphigus?
Bullous pemphigus is a group of autoimmune superficial skin disorders. They may be classified into pemphigus vulgaris, pemphigus foliaceus and paraneoplastic pemphigus, with pemphigus vulgaris being the most common.

Causes
It is thought to be an autoimmune condition where patients produce IgG antibodies against desmoglein (typically types 1 and 3). Desmoglein is an adhesion molecule that is responsible for gluing epidermal cells together.

Symptoms
- Painful superficial blisters – may be erythematous.
- Initially involves the oropharynx but then spreads to other regions such as the face, chest and genital area.
- Nikolsky's sign may be apparent.

Investigations
Punch biopsy with immunofluorescence – visualizes acantholysis.

Bullous pemphigoid

What is bullous pemphigoid?
Bullous pemphigoid is a chronic autoimmune, blistering condition. It is twice as common as bullous pemphigus and tends to present in elderly patients.

Causes
It is thought to be an autoimmune condition in which patients produce IgG antibodies and sometimes also IgE antibodies against specific basement membrane glycoproteins. These are:
- BP180 (most common), aka type XVII collagen.
- BP230, aka plakin.

Symptoms
- Widespread itchy blisters, typically in flexural areas, which heal without scarring (the exception to this is cicatricial pemphigoid, which does scar and also affects the oropharynx).

Investigations
Typically a clinical diagnosis confirmed with punch biopsy followed by immunofluorescence – visualizes IgG and C3 at dermoepidermal junction.

Treatment

Conservative:
- Patient education.
- Drug cessation if responsible for pemphigus-like reaction (e.g. antibiotics [penicillin] and other medications such as captopril and penicillamine).

Medical:
- Oral corticosteroids.
- Immunosuppressants (e.g. azathioprine and methotrexate)
- Plasmapheresis considered in refractory cases.

Complications
- Sepsis.
- Side effects associated with long-term steroid use.

Treatment

Conservative:
- Patient education.
- Drug cessation if responsible for pemphigoid-like reaction (e.g. furosemide and penicillamine).

Medical:
- Topical treatments – steroids in moderate cases.
- Oral corticosteroids.
- Immunosuppressants (e.g. azathioprine and methotrexate).
- Antibiotics if superadded infection present.

Complications
- Usually a self-limiting condition that remits after 1–2 years.
- Superadded infection.
- Side effects associated with long-term steroid or immunosuppressant use.

Map 7.7 Bullous disorders

Map 7.8 Acne vulgaris

What is acne vulgaris?

Acne vulgaris is a common condition that results in a series of skin lesions ranging from comeodomes to pustules, papules and scarring. It may be classified as mild, moderate or severe.

- Mild – comeodomes (open and closed), some papules, some pustules.
- Moderate – increasing number of papules and pustules, mild scarring.
- Severe – comeodomes, papules, pustules plus more extensive scarring and nodular abscesses.

Acne fulminans is a rare but very severe form of acne seen exclusively in adolescent males. It is caused by an immune reaction to *Propionobacterium acnes*.

Causes

Follicular keratinization, seborrhoea and colonization of the pilosebaceous unit with *P. acnes* are central to the development of acne skin lesions.

Research has shown that hormonal factors and genetic components may also play a role since they provide optimal conditions for the growth of *P. acnes* as well as impacting on the subsequent inflammatory reaction.

Exacerbating factors include:

- Cosmetics – particularly oily creams.
- Certain clothing (e.g. high collared shirts)
- Excessive sweating.
- Excessive androgen production (e.g. polycystic ovary syndrome [PCOS]).

Symptoms

All or some of the following lesions may be present:

- Comeodomes.
- Papules.
- Pustules.
- Cysts.
- Pseudocysts.
- Scarring (ice pick scarring).
- Excoriations.
- Erythematous or pigmented macules.

Investigations

Usually a clinical diagnosis; however, in some cases if hyperandrogenism is suspected in females, further tests should be undertaken. (See Map 3.5 [PCOS], p. 84.)

MAP 7.8. **Acne vulgaris**

Treatment

Conservative:
- Patient education.
- Advice regarding skin hygiene.

Medical:
- Mild: blackheads and whiteheads:
  ○ Topical retinoid (e.g. isotretinoin).
  ○ Benzoyl peroxide.
  ○ Consider combined oral contraceptive pill (COCP).
- Moderate: papules and pustules:
  ○ Topical antibiotic with topical retinoid or benzoyl peroxide.
  ○ Oral antibiotic (e.g. lymecycline combined with topical agent).
  ○ Consider COCP.
- Severe: papulopustular with nodules +/- scarring:
  ○ Refer to dermatology for treatment with isotretinoin.
  ○ Provide moderate level acne management while waiting for referral.
  ○ Consider COCP, specifically Dianette.

Complications
- Scarring.
- Psychological (e.g. depression).
- Side effects of treatment (e.g. isotretinoin – cheilitis, increased risk of sunburn, teratogenic, myalgia).

Map 7.8. Acne vulgaris

Map 7.9. Rosacea

What is rosacea?

Rosacea is a chronic inflammatory erythematous dermatosis typically involving the central face. It is more common in women and generally affects those aged 30–60 years.

Causes

The exact cause of rosacea is unknown but it is thought to involve both genetic and environmental factors. Potential influencing factors include:

- Skin type – more common in fair skinned individuals with Celtic origin.
- High levels of cathelicidins (antimicrobial peptides).
- Vasodilation of blood vessels influencing hyperplasia of the sebaceous glands.
- Involvement of matrix metalloproteinases (e.g. elastase and collagenase).

Exacerbating factors include:

- Cosmetics – particularly oily creams.
- Spicy foods.
- Alcohol.
- Heat (e.g. hot showers or hot rooms).
- UV exposure.
- Topical steroids.

Symptoms

All or some of the following lesions may be present:

- Dome shaped papules +/– pustules.
- Facial flushing.
- Telangiectasia.
- Dry and sensitive skin.
- Sebaceous hyperplasia.
- Rhinophyma (whiskey nose).
- Blepharophyma.

Investigations

This is a clinical diagnosis. If a skin biopsy is performed, it will demonstrate vascular and chronic inflammatory changes.

MAP 7.9. Rosacea

Treatment

Conservative:
- Patient education.
- Advice to avoid exacerbating factors.

Medical:
- **Mild:**
  - Topical metronidazole (1st line).
  - Azelaic acid (alternative).
- **Moderate – severe:**
  - Oral tetracyclines or erythromycin.
- **Ocular rosacea:**
  - Ocular lubricants.
  - Oral tetracyclines.

Complications
- Psychological (e.g. depression).
- Ocular rosacea.

Map 7.9. Rosacea

Map 7.10. Alopecia areata

What is alopecia areata?

Hair growth consists of four stages:

1. Anagen – the growth phase.
2. Catagen – the involution phase.
3. Telogen – the resting phase.
4. Release – the release of the hair shaft.

Alopecia areata is a chronic relapsing autoimmune condition where the anagen phase is prematurely arrested. It is a localized non-scarring alopecia. Broadly speaking, alopecia may be defined as diffuse non-scarring, localized scarring, and scarring. Each category has a different cause:

- Diffuse non-scarring: drug induced, metabolic.
- Localized scarring: alopecia areata, trauma, ringworm.
- Scarring: trauma (burns), lichen planus, discoid lupus.

Causes

The exact cause and mechanism of alopecia areata is unknown. In some cases the condition may be triggered by trauma, stress or viral infection. Those with a first-degree relative suffering with alopecia areata are more likely to be affected.

Symptoms

Hair loss may involve the scalp, eyebrows, eyelashes or beard.

- Circular regions of hair loss.
- Non-scarring.
- Exclamation mark hairs.
- Nail changes are apparent in 10–15% of patients and include Beau's lines, onycholysis and koilonychia.

Investigations

Usually a clinical diagnosis. Trichoscopy is used to examine the hair and scalp.

MAP 7.10. Alopecia areata

Treatment

Conservative:

- Patient education.
- Assess the extent of hair loss using scales such as the Lugwig Scale and the Norwood Scale.
- Consider the use of wigs or partial wigs.

Medical:

- Evidence of hair regrowth:
  - No treatment.
- No hair regrowth and <50% hair loss:
  - Discuss watchful waiting and patient preference.
  - If treatment preferred, refer to dermatology where treatment with intralesional corticosteroids may be commenced.
- No hair regrowth and >50% hair loss:
  - Dermatology referral where topical immunotherapy may be commenced.

Complications

- Psychological (e.g. depression).
- Increased risk of other autoimmune conditions (e.g. diabetes and thyroid disease).

Map 7.10. Alopecia areata

Table 7.1 Viral skin infections

TABLE 7.1. **Viral skin infections.**

Disease	Cause	Symptoms	Investigations	Treatment	Complications
Herpes simplex virus (HSV)	Type 1: HSV type 1 Type 2: HSV type 2 Spread via direct contact as well as droplet spread. May reactivate with triggering factors such as stress and trauma	Both forms of HSV may present with a burning or tingling sensation before the outbreak of visual lesions Type 1: perioral lesions – painful vesicles and ulcers. May manifest as herpetic whitlow on infected finger Type 2: penile lesions, vulvovaginitis, anal lesions	Culture/PCR of viral swab	• Aciclovir • Valaciclovir • Famciclovir	• Encephalitis • Ocular infection • Eczema herpeticum • Recurrent erythema multiforme

| Herpes zoster (shingles) | Varicella zoster virus (VZV) Initial infection causes chickenpox. This remains dormant in a sensory root ganglion. When reactivated, shingles occurs | Pain and paraesthesia develop along a dermal distribution up to 5 days before the onset of vesicle development. These vesicles eventually crust over | • Usually a clinical diagnosis
• VZV specific IgM antibody
• Electron microscopy | • Antiviral agent: aciclovir should be given within 72 hours of rash onset
• Analgesia: Mild to moderate – paracetamol alone or in combination with an NSAID or codeine. Severe – if the above methods have failed and pain is severe, consider amitriptyline or pregabalin | • Scarring
• Post-herpetic neuralgia
• Ramsay Hunt syndrome (cranial nerve VII involvement)
• Zoster ophthalmicus (ophthalmic division of the trigeminal nerve affected) |

Continued overleaf

Table 7.1 Viral skin infections

Table 7.1: Viral skin infections

TABLE 7.1: **Viral skin infections** (*continued*).

Disease	Cause	Symptoms	Investigations	Treatment	Complications

Viral warts	Human papillomavirus (HPV) – a double-stranded DNA virus. There are many different types involved with wart formation in different regions of the body:
	
	• Type 1: plantar warts
	• Type 2: plantar warts and common warts
	• Type 4: common warts
	• Types 6 & 11: anogenital warts
	• Type 16: oropharyngeal cancer
	• Type 16 & 18: cervical cancer
		Dome-shaped papules/nodules with an irregular papilliferous surface	• Clinical diagnosis
			• Microscopy – hyperkeratotic epidermis
			• Cervical smear with liquid-based cytology – for cervical HPV
				• HPV vaccination programme aiming to reduce the prevalence of cervical cancer
				• For warts:
				  ○ Salicylic acid
				  ○ Imiquimod cream
				  ○ Cryotherapy with liquid nitrogen
					• Pain (e.g. plantar wart affecting gait cycle)
					• Spread
					• Local infection
					• Malignant change

TABLE 7.2. **Parasitic skin infections.**

Disease	Cause	Symptoms	Investigations	Treatment	Complications
Head lice	*Pediculosis humanus capitis*	• May be asymptomatic • Itching	Visualization of infestation. A fine toothcomb is often used	Insecticidal shampoo containing permethrin or malathion. Treat household members and close contacts if infested	Infection secondary to scratching
Scabies	*Sarcoptes scabiei*	• Itching • Small papules where the mite has burrowed beneath the skin – often at the webs of fingers, the wrist and in the genital region • Linear tracks of the burrowing mite	Clinical diagnosis Mite may be visualized on dermatoscopy	• Permethrin or malathion should be applied to the entire body except the face • All household members and close contacts require treatment • Bed linen etc. requires thorough washing on high heat	Norwegian crusted scabies in immunosuppressed patients

Table 7.2. Parasitic skin infections

Table 7.3: Bacterial skin infections

TABLE 7.3. **Bacterial skin infections.**

Disease	Cause	Symptoms	Investigations	Treatment	Complications
Impetigo	*Staphylococcus aureus* (commonest) Streptococci	• Erythematous erosions with yellow crusting	Bacterial swabs	• Topical fucidin cream • Flucloxacillin (*S. aureus*) • Penicillin (streptococci) • Erythromycin if allergic to penicillin	• Scarring • Post-streptococcal glomerulonephritis • Scarlet fever • Septicaemia • Staphylococcal scalded skin syndrome
Cellulitis	Beta-haemolytic streptococci *Staphylococcus aureus*	• Tenderness on palpation • Erythematous lesion • Cardinal signs of inflammation • Lymphadenopathy • Fever • Malaise	Often a clinical diagnosis. Follow local hospital guidelines and take blood cultures	• Flucloxacillin (*S. aureus*) • Penicillin (streptococci) • Erythromycin if allergic to penicillin	• Septicaemia • Abscess formation – requires surgical drainage • Toxic shock-like syndrome

Gas gangrene	*Clostridium perfringens*	• Symptoms occur at the site of trauma • Inflammation • Pain • Induration • In advanced disease – crepitus felt in muscle and distal pulses are lost	• Swabs – Gram stain • Blood tests – FBC, WCC, LDH, blood cultures, biochemistry profile • Imaging – radiography and CT scanning	• Wound debridement • Skin grafting may be required in severe cases • Penicillin	• Scarring – may require reconstructive surgery • Multi-organ failure
Leprosy (Hansen's disease)	*Mycobacterium leprae*, an intracellular acid–fast bacillus (granulomatous disease)	• Skin lesions – erythematous or hypopigmented • Peripheral nerve involvement – motor weakness and sensory impairment • Saddle nose • Loss of digits/limbs due to secondary infections There are three different forms of leprosy: • Tuberculoid: mildest form • Lepromatous: most severe form and very contagious • Borderline: mixed picture of tuberculoid and lepromatous forms	Skin biopsy – acid–fast bacillus	• Dapsone • Rifampicin	• Scarring and disfiguration • Male infertility and erectile dysfunction • Glaucoma • Kidney failure • Permanent peripheral nerve injury

Table 7.3: Bacterial skin infections

Table 7.4 Fungal skin infections

TABLE 7.4 **Fungal skin infections.**

Disease	Cause	Symptoms	Investigations	Treatment	Complications
Candidiasis	*Candida albicans*, a commensal yeast Risk factors include anything that causes immuno-suppression, for example: • HIV • Diabetes • Cancer • Anaemia	Depends on location: 1. Skin – sore, itchy skin. Commonly affects flexures, where lesions appear erythematous 2. Oral candidiasis – pain, difficulty eating/swallowing, altered taste, white pseudomembrane may be present 3. Candidal oesophagitis – odynophagia, weight loss 4. Balanitis – penile itching and soreness, dysuria 5. Vulvovaginal candidiasis – vulval itching and soreness, vaginal discharge, dysuria, superficial dyspareunia	Tends to be a clinical diagnosis but it is important to swab the lesion if there is any uncertainty, if there is a superadded bacterial infection or if the patient is immunocompro-mised.	1. Skin: ○ Adult, not immunocompromised – topical imidazole ○ Child, not immunocompromised – topical clotrimazole, miconazole, econazole ○ Adult, immunocompromised – oral fluconazole ○ Child, immunocompromised – seek specialist advice, consider oral fluconazole 2. Oral: ○ Adults and children, not immunocompromised – miconazole gel or nystatin suspension ○ Adults, immunocompromised – oral fluconazole 3. Candidal oesophagitis: ○ Oral fluconazole 4. Balanitis: ○ Adults – imidazole cream (or oral fluconazole, single dose for those over 16 years) ○ Children – a topical imidazole cream 5. Vulvovaginal candidiasis ○ Adults, not immunocompromised – intravaginal fluconazole or itraconazole. Vulval symptoms may be treated with a topical imidazole cream. If severe, clotrimazole cream may be used ○ Adults, immunocompromised – oral fluconazole or itraconazole	• Superadded infection • Specific complications depending on location; for example, odynophagia or superficial dyspareunia

| Ringworm | Dermato-phyte fungi | 1. Body and groin – tinea cruris
○ Erythematous, flat or potentially mildly raised ring shaped lesions with a central clearing
2. Scalp – tinea capitis
○ Itching
○ Scalp scarring
○ Patchy hair loss
3. Foot – tinea pedis
○ Typical white, cracked interdigital lesions | 1. Body and groin – tinea cruris
○ Usually a clinical diagnosis but if there is any doubt, send a sample for microscopy and culture
2. Scalp – tinea capitis
○ Scalp scraping for microscopy and culture
3. Foot – tinea pedis
○ Usually a clinical diagnosis but if there is any doubt, send a sample for microscopy and culture | 1. Body and groin – tinea cruris
○ Mild – topical antifungal creams
○ Severe – oral antifungal agents
2. Scalp – tinea capitis
○ Adults – oral antifungals
○ Children – consider oral antifungals or refer to specialist
○ If kerion present – refer to dermatology
3. Foot – tinea pedis
○ Mild – topical clotrimazole, miconazole or econazole
○ Severe – oral antifungal agents | • Potentially serious and refractory cases in those who are immuno-compromised |

Table 7.4. Fungal skin infections

TABLE 7.5. **Skin lumps.**

Disease	Cause	Symptoms	Investigations	Treatment	Complications
Seborrhoeic keratosis	Proliferation of the basal layer of epidermis. Increased risk with sun exposure and age	• Flat/raised papules/plaques • Wart-like, pedunculated yellow-brown appearance • Lesion may itch and bleed • Typically arises on the trunk	• Clinical diagnosis • Dermatoscopy may be useful	• Cryotherapy • Curettage	Skin cancer may arise from or be difficult to distinguish from these lesions
Solar keratosis	Scaly plaques that occur as a result of UVB damage	• Well-demarcated yellow–brown, erythematous hyperkeratotic scaly lesion • Lesion may itch and bleed	• Clinical diagnosis • Dermatoscopy may be useful • Biopsy may be used to rule out squamous cell carcinoma	• Cryotherapy • Curettage • Creams – 5-fluorouracil (cytotoxic), imiquimod	Squamous cell carcinoma
Dermatofibroma	A benign nodule that typically arises on the lower leg but may arise elsewhere. More common in women than in men	• Firm, pigmented nodules usually present on the lower leg • Between 1 and 15 in number • Mobile over subcutaneous tissue • Nodule(s) may be itchy or asymptomatic	• Clinical diagnosis • Dermatoscopy may be useful • Biopsy taken if there is any uncertainty concerning diagnosis	Only remove if causing trouble to patients	Bleeding if traumatized

Haemangioma	This is a benign condition of cutaneous blood vessels caused by arteriovenous malformation or abnormal vessel proliferation. There are many different types. Some examples are listed below: 1. Strawberry naevus – this resolves with time. Treatment is generally not required unless superadded infection occurs or it develops in a problematic region (e.g. the eyelid) 2. Port-wine stain – associated with Sturge–Weber syndrome 3. Cavernous haemangioma – associated with Kasabach–Merritt syndrome 4. Pyogenic granuloma – follows trauma	• Depends on the type of haemangioma • Lesions may be singular but in some cases multiple • The lesions are erythematous and may be flat or raised • There may be thickening of the overlying epidermis	• Usually a clinical diagnosis • USS is used to investigate deep infantile haemangiomas • MRI and angiography may be required in more complex cases	• Sometimes no treatment is required • Propanolol • Compressive therapy • Laser therapy • Intralesional steroid injections	• Psychological implications (e.g. depression) • Ulceration • Bleeding

Continued overleaf

Table 7.5 Skin lumps

TABLE 7.5. **Skin lumps** (*continued*).

Disease	Cause	Symptoms	Investigations	Treatment	Complications
Lipoma	Benign slow growing tumour comprised of lobulated fat cells. A thin fibrous capsule encases the tumour. It affects males and females equally; however, multiple lesions are more common in men	Smooth, soft, rubbery swelling ~2–10 cm in diameter	• Usually a clinical diagnosis • Skin biopsy may be performed if there is any doubt of the diagnosis. This will visualize a thin fibrous capsule and capillaries with fibrous strands	Often treatment is not required. If problematic, surgical excision may be required	Interference with adjacent muscle movement
Epidermoid cyst	Epithelium lined cavity filled with semi-solid material. Mostly occur in hair bearing areas	Dermal lump with characteristic central punctum	Usually a clinical diagnosis	Surgical excision	• Rupture • Infection • Skin cancer
Dermoid cyst	Cyst arising from epidermal cells, lined by squamous epithelium	Smooth, soft, rubbery swelling. Two different types: 1. Implantation cysts – arise following trauma 2. Congenital cysts – arise from embryonic fusion sites	Usually a clinical diagnosis	Surgical excision	Rupture Infection Torsion

Table 7.5. Skin lumps

Table 7.6. Skin tumours

TABLE 7.6. **Skin tumours. Risk factors include: skin type 1, history of sun burn/sun exposure (particularly in childhood), precancerous skin lesions, personal or family history of skin cancer, radiation exposure, multiple moles, genetics – familial dysplastic naevus syndrome (chromosome 1).**

Disease	Cause	Symptoms	Investigations	Treatment	Complications
Basal cell carcinoma	Sun exposure, particularly prevalent in skin type 1 and excessive childhood sun exposure Associated with mutations of the tumour suppressor gene (chromosome 9)	Depends on the type of basal cell carcinoma: 1. Nodular type: commonest, pigmented nodule with telangiectasia 2. Superficial type: irregular pigmented plaques 3. Morphoeic type: flesh coloured plaques	• Dermatoscopy • Excision biopsy	Surgical excision	Local invasion – rodent ulcer
Squamous cell carcinoma	Refer to above risk factors	A locally invasive tumour that typically ulcerates with rolled edges. Two types: 1. Bowen's disease – squamous cell carcinoma in situ 2. Keratoacanthoma – central keratin plug	• Dermatoscopy • Excision biopsy	• Bowen's disease – cryotherapy, curettage or topical 5-fluorouracil • Surgical excision	Spread to lymph nodes

| Malignant melanoma | Refer to above risk factors | Remember to assess the lesion **ABCDE**, which directly relates to the symptoms of this malignancy:

A – Asymmetrical lesion
B – Borders are irregular
C – Colour has changed
D – Diameter increased
E – Evolving lesion

The lesion may also itch and bleed | • Dermatoscopy
• Assessment using Clark levels and Breslow's thickness

Clark levels:
1. Melanoma in situ
2. Invasion of the papillary dermis
3. Invasion into the junction of the papillary and reticular dermis
4. Invasion of the reticular dermis
5. Invasion of the subcutaneous fat

Breslow's thickness:
Thin: <1 mm
Intermediate: 1–4 mm
Thick: >4 mm | • Wide surgical excision
• If metastasis, then chemotherapy and radiotherapy is required | • Metastasis
• Death |

Table 7.6: Skin tumours

Table 8.1a. General complications of fractures

Fractures

There are many different types of fracture and they may be defined (1) by location, (2) as open (compound) or closed, (3) as intra- or extra-articular, (4) as displaced or not displaced, (5) by type: (a) complex – comminuted, segmental, (b) non-complex – transverse, oblique, spiral, avulsion etc., (c) specific (e.g. greenstick), and (6) by disease involvement (e.g. osteoporosis).

Fractures must be further assessed using radiography, and a description of impaction, angulation and translocation must be reported. The many complications associated with fractures are outlined below.

TABLE 8.1a. **General complications of fractures.**

Complication	Comments
General	• Haemorrhage • Shock • Infection • Fat embolus resulting in pulmonary embolism and respiratory distress syndrome • Rhabdomyolysis
Associated with prolonged bed rest	• Deep vein thrombosis and pulmonary embolism • Pressure sores • Muscle wasting • Infection

Associated with plaster casts	• Remember as **SPAN:**
	  S – **S**tiffness
	  P – **P**ressure
	  A – **A**llergy
	  N – **N**erve and circulatory disturbance

Associated with anaesthesia	• Anaphylaxis • Aspiration

TABLE 8.1b Specific complications of fractures.

Complication	Comments
Immediate	<ul><li>Haemorrhage</li><li>Neurovascular complications</li></ul>
Early	<ul><li>Infection</li><li>Compartment syndrome:<ul><li>Fractures cause swelling, which increases the pressure within the compartment. This results in decreased capillary blood flow. Ischaemia develops when capillary pressure is less than that of the compartment pressure. Irreversible change results after 6 hours</li><li>Symptoms include pain, which is out of proportion with presenting symptoms. This pain is present/worsened on passive stretching. Paraesthesia and tightness may also be present</li></ul></li></ul>
Late	<ul><li>Malunion<ul><li>Two different forms:<ol><li>Hypertrophic – plenty of new bone growth but these fail to unite</li><li>Atrophic – lack of new bone growth. Osteopenic in appearance</li></ol></li></ul></li><li>Avascular necrosis</li><li>Complex regional pain syndrome<ul><li>Two different forms:<ol><li>No underlying nerve problem</li><li>Underlying, demonstrable nerve problem</li></ol></li></ul></li><li>Myositis ossificans – calcification of the soft tissues, which occurs after surgery or injury</li><li>Growth disturbance – occurs after damage to the growth plate. This is described using the Salter-Harris classification. Remember as **SALT C**: **S** – Separate (fracture occurs through the growth plate) **A** – Above (above the growth plate. Most common type) **L** – Lower (below the growth plate) **T** – Through (both upper and lower. Commonest cause of premature growth arrest) **C** – Crushed physis (worst injury)</li></ul>

Table 8.1b Specific complications of fractures

Map 8.1. Neck pathology

Cervical spondylosis

What is cervical spondylosis?
Degenerative arthritis of the cervical vertebrae. There is increased risk with age.

Causes
- Osteoarthritis resulting in bony spurs. This may result in a cervical radiculopathy or myelopathy.
- Trauma.

Symptoms
- May be asymptomatic.
- Reduced range of movement.
- Pain.
- Paraesthesia following a dermatomal distribution.

Investigations
- Thorough physical examination.
- Lhermitte's sign.
- Radiology – CT/MRI.

Treatment
- Conservative: physiotherapy.
- Medical: NSAIDs, codeine etc.; follow WHO analgesic ladder.
- Surgical: anterior cervical discectomy, cervical laminectomy.

Complications
- Vertebrobasilar insufficiency.

Cervical spondylolisthesis

What is cervical spondylolisthesis?
This is when a superiorly located cervical vertebra is displaced anteriorly relative to the vertebra below. This may narrow the vertebral canal and results in deformity.

Causes
- Congenital: failure of ondontoid process fusion.
- Trauma: results in instability.
- Softening of the transverse ligament due to inflammation.

Symptoms
- Pain – may be radicular or may radiate between the shoulder blades and to the back of the head.

Investigations
- Thorough physical examination.
- Radiology: CT/MRI.
- Meyerding grading system – describes percentage slippage.

Treatment
- Conservative: physiotherapy.
- Medical: NSAIDs, codeine etc.; follow WHO analgesic ladder. Consider corticosteroid injections.
- Surgical: microdiscectomy, hemilaminectomy, anterior cervical discectomy +/– fusion.

MAP 8.1. **Neck pathology**

Cervical disc prolapse

What is a cervical disc prolapse?

This occurs when the nucleus pulposus herniates through a tear in the annulus fibrosus. Typically affects C5/6 and C6/7 since these are the most mobile segments. Prolapses may be central or lateral.

Symptoms

- Brachalgia with associated radiculopathy.
- Pain, paraesthsia, weakness.

Investigations

- Thorough physical examination.
- Radiology – MRI.

Treatment

Depends on the extent of the prolapse and the presence or absence of neurological symptoms.

- Mild – no neurological symptoms. Physiotherapy and analgesia may suffice.
- Moderate – only radicular symptoms. Surgery may be required (e.g. discectomy or laminectomy).
- Severe – urgent surgical decompression.

Map 8.2. Shoulder pathology

MAP 8.2. **Shoulder pathology**

Shoulder dislocation

What is a shoulder dislocation?
This is when there is a loss of congruity between the head of the humerus and the glenoid fossa. There are two types – anterior and posterior.

Causes
- Anterior – commonest. Trauma. Increased risk in those with connective tissue disorders or those with prior shoulder dislocations.
- Posterior – rare. Seizures and electrocution.

Symptoms
- Pain.
- Decreased range of movement.
- Anterior – humeral head is prominent and held in an abducted, externally rotated position.

Rotator cuff tears

What are rotator cuff tears?
The rotator cuff comprises four tendons and muscles that aim to provide stability to the highly mobile shoulder joint. The four muscles (remembered as **SITS**) are the **S**upraspinatus (most commonly torn), **I**nfraspinatus, **T**eres minor and **S**ubscapularis. Further important anatomical details about these muscles are provided below:

Muscle	Action	Innervation	Specific test
Supraspinatus	Abducts humerus	Suprascapular nerve (C5)	Empty beer can test (eliminates deltoid)
Infraspinatus	Externally rotates humerus	Suprascapular nerve (C5–6)	Resisted external rotation
Teres minor	Externally rotates humerus	Axillary nerve (C5)	-
Subscapularis	Internally rotates humerus	Upper and lower subscapular nerve (C5–6)	Lift-off test

Investigations

- Radiology – x-ray (lateral and AP views).

Treatment

- Closed reduction and sling immobilization.
- Adequate analgesia.

Complications

- Axillary nerve or artery damage.
- Damage to the brachial plexus.
- Increased risk of recurrence.
- Specific lesions:
  - Bankart lesion: avulsion of antero-inferior glenoid labrum.
  - Hill–Sachs lesion: indentation fracture of the posterolateral humeral head.

Causes

- Degeneration.
- Trauma.
- Weight lifting.

Symptoms

- Partial tears result in a painful arc syndrome.
- Complete tears limit shoulder abduction.
- Pain to a variable degree depending on the significance of the tear.
- Shoulder tenderness on palpation.
- Weakness.

Investigations

- Thorough examination with specific tests as outlined in Table above.
- Radiology – x-ray, MRI.

Treatment

- Conservative: rest and physiotherapy.
- Medical: adequate pain relief.
- Surgical: arthroscopy +/– repair if indicated.

Complications

- Decreased range of movement, which may inhibit daily activities such as getting dressed.
- Complications associated with surgery include general risks from anaesthesia and infection as well as specific complications such as damage to the axillary nerve.

Continued overleaf

Map 8.2. Shoulder pathology

Map 8.2. Shoulder pathology

MAP 8.2. **Shoulder pathology** (*continued*)

Adhesive capsulitis

What is adhesive capsulitis?

Adhesive capsulitis is also known as frozen shoulder. Typically the pathology encompasses three phases:

1. Pain with freezing.
2. Thawing.
3. Resolution – may take up to and possibly more than 2 years.

Causes

- The exact aetiology of this condition is unknown but it is linked to trauma and past shoulder surgery.

Risk factors

- Increased age.
- Female.
- Diabetes mellitus.
- Rheumatoid arthritis.

Symptoms

- Pain – on active and passive movement.
- Restricted range on movement – actively and passively. External rotation is often affected first.
- Often no movement at the glenohumeral joint.
- Difficulty sleeping on the affected side.

Investigations

- Thorough physical examination.
- Radiology: USS and MRI.

Treatment

- Conservative: physiotherapy.
- Medical: adequate analgesia, steroid injections.
- Surgery: only performed in severe cases (e.g. capsular release via arthroscopy).

Complications

- Stiffness.
- Loss of function.

FIGURE 8.1. **The brachial plexus**

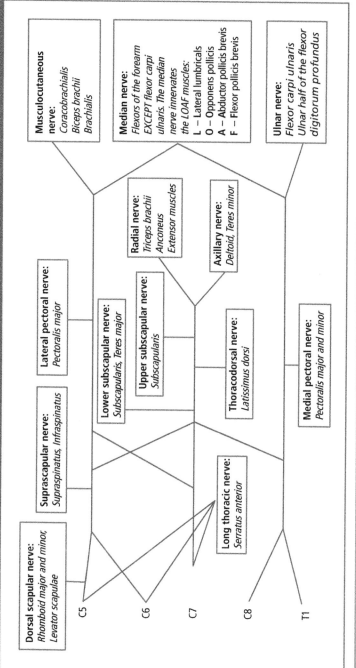

Dorsal scapular nerve:
Rhomboid major and minor,
Levator scapulae

Suprascapular nerve:
Supraspinatus, Infraspinatus

Lateral pectoral nerve:
Pectoralis major

Musculocutaneous nerve:
Coracobrachialis
Biceps brachii
Brachialis

Lower subscapular nerve:
Subscapularis, Teres major

Upper subscapular nerve:
Subscapularis

Radial nerve:
Triceps brachii
Anconeus
Extensor muscles

Median nerve:
Flexors of the forearm
EXCEPT flexor carpi
ulnaris. The median
nerve innervates
the LOAF muscles:
L – Lateral lumbricals
O – Opponens pollicis
A – Abductor pollicis brevis
F – Flexor pollicis brevis

Axillary nerve:
Deltoid, Teres minor

Thoracodorsal nerve:
Latissimus dorsi

Long thoracic nerve:
Serratus anterior

Medial pectoral nerve:
Pectoralis major and minor

Ulnar nerve:
Flexor carpi ulnaris
Ulnar half of the flexor
digitorum profundus

C5

C6

C7

C8

T1

Figure 8.1. The brachial plexus

Map 8.3. Arthritis

MAP 8.3. **Arthritis**

Rheumatoid arthritis

What is rheumatoid arthritis (RA)?

This is a chronic, autoimmune type III hypersensitivity reaction that principally affects the synovium but may also affect other organs. Joint involvement is characterized by symmetrical deformation with pain that is worse in the morning. This condition is associated with HLA-DR4 and HLA-DR1.

Cause

The exact cause of RA is unknown, but it is thought to involve a type III hypersensitivity reaction.

Signs and symptoms

- Hands – Z deformity, boutonnière deformity, swan neck deformity, ulnar deviation, subluxation of the fingers, Raynaud's association.
- Wrist – carpal tunnel syndrome.
- Feet – subluxation of the toes, hammer toe deformity.
- Skin – rheumatoid nodule, vasculitis.
- Cardiovascular – atherosclerosis is increased in RA.
- Respiratory – pulmonary fibrosis.
- Bones – osteoporosis.
- Pain and stiffness.

Osteoarthritis

What is osteoarthritis (OA)?

This is a degenerative arthritis affecting synovial joints and is characterized by cartilage degeneration, associated response of the periarticular tissue and pain that is typically worse at the end of the day.

Cause

Damage to the joints and general wear and tear of the joint over time is thought to be the primary cause of OA. There are certain factors that increase the risk of OA such as:

- Increased age.
- Obesity.
- Trauma to the joint.
- Conditions such as haemochromatosis and Ehlers–Danlos syndrome.

Signs and symptoms

- Pain and stiffness.
- Swelling around joint involved.
- Crepitus.
- Heberden's nodes (distal interphalangeal joints).
- Bouchard's nodes (proximal interphalangeal joints).

Investigations

- Bloods:
  - 80% test positive for rheumatoid factor.
  - ESR and CRP raised.
  - Cyclic citrullinated peptide. If positive, suggestive of erosive disease.
- Radiology: radiological signs of RA are visualized on plain film:
  - Bony erosion, subluxation, carpal instability.
  - Involvement of metacarpo- and metatarsophalangeal joints.
  - Periarticular osteoporosis.

Treatment

- Conservative: patient education. Encourage exercise. Refer to physiotherapy and assess activities of daily living (ADLs).
- Medical: glucocorticoids, disease modifying antirheumatic drugs (DMARDs) (e.g. gold salts, methotrexate, sulphasalazine). Anticytokine therapies may be considered in patients intolerant to methotrexate.
- Surgery: excision arthroplasty or replacement may be considered in severely affected joints.

Complications

- Carpal tunnel syndrome.
- Pericarditis.
- Sjögren's syndrome.
- Cervical myopathy.
- Tendon rupture.

Investigations

- Bloods: usually not diagnostic but may be relevant when OA is related to another condition such as haemochromatosis.
- Radiology: radiological signs (LOSS):
  - L – Loss of joint space
  - O – Osteophytes
  - S – Subchondral cysts
  - S – Sclerosis

Treatment

- Conservative: patient education. Encourage exercise and weight loss.
- Medical: analgesia (e.g. paracetamol or NSAIDs). Gels such as capsaicin may be useful. Steroid injections.
- Surgical: arthroplasty.

Complications

- Increased risk of gout.
- Chondrocalcinosis.

Map 8.3. Arthritis

Map 8.4. Elbow pathology

MAP 8.4: Elbow pathology

Tennis elbow

What is tennis elbow?

Tennis elbow is also known as lateral epicondylitis and is the most common elbow overuse injury. The lateral epicondyle is the origin of the common extensor tendon and in tennis elbow it becomes inflamed and causes elbow pain.

Causes

Tennis elbow is a form of repetitive strain injury (e.g. playing sports such as tennis, squash) or undertaking other activities such as gardening and painting. This results in microrupture/microtears and degenerative changes in the tendon as well as inflammation, particularly at the muscular origin of extensor carpi radialis brevis.

Symptoms

- Aching elbow pain, typically over the lateral epicondyle, which worsens with activity.
- Typically affects the dominant arm.
- Worse during simple daily tasks utilizing extensors, such as lifting a cup of coffee.
- Decreased power grip in affected arm.

Golfer's elbow

What is golfer's elbow?

Golfer's elbow is also known as medial epicondylitis and is a type of elbow overuse injury. The medial epicondyle is the origin of the common flexor tendon and in golfer's elbow it becomes inflamed and causes elbow pain.

Causes

Golfer's elbow is a form of repetitive strain injury (e.g. playing sports such as golf, bowling, baseball, rock climbing) or undertaking other activities such as gardening, painting and using tools like screwdrivers. This results in microrupture/microtears and degenerative changes in the tendon as well as inflammation.

Symptoms

- Aching elbow pain, typically over the medial epicondyle, which worsens with activity.
- Typically affects the dominant arm.
- Worse during simple daily tasks utilizing flexors.
- Decreased power grip in affected arm.

Investigations

- No specific tests or imaging required.
- Clinical diagnosis.
- Golfer's elbow test.

Investigations

- No specific tests or imaging required.
- Clinical diagnosis.
- Mill's test and Cozen's test.

Treatment

- Conservative: usually a self-limiting condition, stop/decrease activity that triggered tennis elbow, ice elbow, utilize an elbow strap, physiotherapy may be required.
- Medical: painkillers (e.g. paracetamol and NSAIDs), local steroid injections if severe and other methods have failed.
- Surgery: only considered if above methods have failed and if pain lasts for up to 4 months.

Complications

- Loss of function.
- Chronic pain.

Treatment

- Conservative: usually a self-limiting condition, stop/decrease activity that triggered golfer's elbow, ice elbow, utilize an elbow strap, physiotherapy may be required.
- Medical: painkillers (e.g. paracetamol and NSAIDs), local steroid injections if severe and other methods have failed.
- Surgery: only considered if above methods have failed and if pain lasts for up to 4 months.

Complications

- Loss of function.
- Chronic pain.
- Associated ulnar neuropathy.

Remember the difference between tennis elbow and golfer's elbow as:

Tennis is played on the Lawn (i.e. Tennis elbow is Lateral epicondylitis)

Golf is played on the Meadow (i.e. Golfer's elbow is Medial epicondylitis)

Map 8.4. Elbow pathology

MAP 8.5. **Hand pathology**

Dupuytren's contracture

What is Dupuytren's contracture?

Dupuytren's contracture is a proliferative fibroplasia of the palmar and digital fascia. Over time this leads to the formation of nodules and cords, which in turn result in finger flexion. The ring finger is most commonly affected.

Causes

The exact cause of this pathology is unknown. It is known that it is more common in males than females as well as in those with a positive family history. It is associated with the following:

- Diabetes mellitus.
- Hepatic cirrhosis.
- Certain drugs (e.g. phenytoin)
- Trauma.

The aggressive form of the disease is called Dupuytren's diathesis and is associated with Peyronie's disease (penile fibromatosis) and Ledderhose's disease (plantar fascia fibromatosis).

Symptoms

- Flexion contracture of the fingers.
- Nodular thickening of palmar fascia and cord development.

de Quervain's syndrome

What is de Quervain's syndrome?

de Quervain's syndrome, also known as washerwoman's sprain, is a stenosing tenosynovitis of the extensor pollicis brevis and the abductor pollicis tendons.

Causes

The exact cause of this condition is unknown but it is associated with overuse/repetitive tasks.

Symptoms

- Wrist pain (radial side), which is worse on movement.

Investigations

- Finkelstein's test – pain on passive ulnar deviation (fist formed over thumb).
- Radiology – x-ray to rule out other conditions such as osteoarthritis.

Treatment

- Conservative: rest and avoidance of precipitating factors.
- Medical: analgesia, steroid injections.
- Surgical: last resort for severe cases – release of first extensor compartment.

Complications

- Decreased range of movement of the wrist.

Stenosing tenosynovitis

What is stenosing tenosynovitis?

This is also known as trigger finger. The flexor tendon sheath narrows due to thickening of the tendon sheath, usually due to trauma. The ring and middle finger are most commonly affected.

Causes
- Typically trauma.
- Associated with diabetes mellitus, rheumatoid arthritis and gout.

Symptoms
- Trapped flexor tendon, usually related to the A1 pulley.
- Digit locked in flexion and must be passively released.

Investigations: clinical diagnosis.

Treatment
- Conservative: immobilization.
- Medical: analgesia, steroid injections.
- Surgery: intractable cases may require surgical release.

Complications
- Related to surgery (e.g. infection, nerve injury, tendon bowstringing).

Continued overleaf

Investigations
- No specific test but can test for underlying associations.
- Perform Hueston's tabletop test.

Treatment
- Surgical – only perform fasciotomy, fasciectomy or dermofasciectomy if contracture is causing functional problems. Physiotherapy and splinting required after treatment.

Complications
- Loss of function.
- Complications associated with surgery (e.g. haematoma formation, nerve injury and recurrence).

Orthopaedics

MAP 8.5. Hand pathology

MAP 8.5. **Hand pathology** (*continued*)

Carpal tunnel syndrome

What is carpal tunnel syndrome?
Carpal tunnel syndrome may be defined as the compression of the median nerve as it passes through the carpal tunnel, beneath the flexor retinaculum. It is more common in females than males.

Causes
Remember as **MEDIAN TRAP**:

M – Myxoedema
E – oEdema
D – Diabetes mellitus
I – Idiopathic
A – Acromegaly
N – Neoplasm

T – Trauma
R – Rheumatoid arthritis
A – Amyloidosis
P – Pregnancy

Symptoms
Remember as **3Ps**
- Pain – in the median nerve distribution, worse at night.

Scaphoid fracture

What is a scaphoid fracture?
The scaphoid is the most commonly fractured wrist bone. The reason this fracture is so important to assess fundamentally rests in the blood supply to this bone. The blood supply enters the distal part of the scaphoid bone and runs proximally. This means that there is a risk of proximal avascular necrosis if fractured.

Causes
- Trauma – typically 'fall on outstretched hand' (FOOSH).

Symptoms
- Pain over the scaphoid bone (i.e. on palpation of the anatomical snuff box).

Investigations
- Radiology – x-ray. Fracture may not be seen initially. If not seen but it is suspected clinically, immobilize in a scaphoid splint and repeat the x-ray in 10 days to 2 weeks.

Treatment
- Scaphoid plaster.

Complications
- Avascular necrosis (proximal third).
- Osteoarthritis.
- Malunion.

- **Paraesthesia** – in the median nerve distribution, relieve by shaking hands.
- **Patch** – on thenar eminence is preserved since the superficial branch of the median nerve supplies this area. Thenar muscle may have wasted in advanced disease.

Investigations
- Usually a clinical diagnosis coupled with a thorough physical examination including specific Tinel's and Phalen's tests.
- Nerve conduction studies – differentiates from cervical spondylosis (C6/7).

Treatment
- Conservative: splinting.
- Medical: steroid injection.
- Surgical: carpal tunnel release.

MAP 8.6. Spinal pathology

MAP 8.6. Spinal pathology

Scoliosis

What is scoliosis?

This is a lateral curvature of the spine that is >10° (Cobb angle). It may be structural or non-structural and broadly speaking there are five different types. Remember as **PONDS**:

P – Postural: non-structural compensatory scoliosis

O – Osteopathic: structural abnormality. Mostly congenital but some cases may be associated with bone disease

N – Neuromuscular: associated with cerebral palsy, Friedreich's ataxia etc.

D – Degenerative: associated with facet joint failure

S – Structural idiopathic: may be subdivided into five types:

1. Thoracolumbar – usually curves to the right
2. Lumbar – usually curves to the left
3. Infantile thoracic – usually curves to the left
4. Adolescent thoracic – usually curves to the right
5. Double major – two curves in each direction

Causes

See above. Remember to ask about family history and pregnancy.

Symptoms

- Cosmetic deformity.

Kyphosis

What is kyphosis?

This is an exaggerated anterior curvature of the thoracic spine. Kyphosis may be classified as fixed, as in ankylosing spondylitis, or mobile as in postural kyphosis. It may also be defined related to shape (i.e. regular or angular [gibbus]).

There are many different types of kyphosis. Remember as **PONDS**:

P – Postural – more common in adolescent girls

O – Osteoporotic

N – Neuromuscular

D – Degenerative

S – Scheuermann's disease – also known as spinal osteochondrosis. Defined as kyphosis >40° and wedging of individual vertebra of 5° (since the vertebra grows more thickly posteriorly than anteriorly)

Causes

Causes include:

- Infection – TB, polio.
- Malignancy.
- Bone disease – osteoporosis, Paget's disease.
- Ankylosing spondylitis.
- Calvé's disease.

- Aching, but not severe, pain. If pain is very severe, then must exclude spinal tumours/osteoid osteomas.

Investigations
- Thorough spinal examination.
- Radiology – x-ray (AP and lateral views) and Cobb angle measurement.
- Investigations concerning an underlying cause if suspected.

Treatment
- Conservative: physiotherapy, exercise (particularly swimming), brace – Boston or Milwaukee.
- Medical: adequate analgesia.
- Surgical: only in severe cases.

Complications
- Psychological implications (e.g. depression).
- Restrictive lung disease.
- Cardiac complications.
- Nerve compression.

Symptoms
- Cosmetic deformity.
- Aching, but not severe, pain. If pain is very severe, then must exclude spinal tumours/osteoid osteomas.
- Symptoms of underlying condition.

Investigations
- Thorough spinal examination.
- Radiology – x-ray (AP and lateral views) and Cobb angle measurement.
- Investigations concerning an underlying cause if suspected.

Treatment
- Conservative: physiotherapy, exercise, particularly swimming.
- Medical: adequate analgesia.
- Surgery: only in severe cases.

Complications
- Psychological implications (e.g. depression)
- Restrictive lung disease.
- Cardiac complications.
- Cord compression.
- Paraplegia.

Continued overleaf

MAP 8.6. Spinal pathology

MAP 8.6. **Spinal pathology** (*continued*)

Spinal stenosis

What is spinal stenosis?
This is a narrowing of the spinal canal, which results in compression of the spinal cord and corresponding nerves.

Causes
- Arthritis.
- Age.
- Trauma.
- Space-occupying lesion.
- Spondylolisthesis.

Symptoms
- Unilateral or bilateral leg pain +/– back pain that is usually of gradual onset.
- Numbness and weakness that worsens with walking.
- Pain relieved by sitting and leaning forwards.

Investigations
- Thorough physical examination.
- Radiology – MRI.

Ankylosing spondylitis

What is ankylosing spondylitis?
This is a chronic inflammatory disease of the spine and sacroiliac joints. There is predominance in young males and the condition is associated with HLA-B27 (positive in 95%).

Causes
The exact cause and pathophysiology of this condition are unknown. However, it is thought to be associated with HLA-B27.

Signs and symptoms
Symptoms improve with exercise.
- Question mark posture.
- Pain and stiffness.
- Extra-articular features:
  Iritis.
  Aortitis.
  Apical pulmonary fibrosis.
  Amyloidosis (secondary).
  Cardiac conduction defects.
- Specific spinal symptoms:
  Bamboo spine – due to calcification of ligaments.
  Low back pain and stiffness.
  Loss of lumbar lordosis.
  Compensatory fixed kyphosis.

MAP 8.6. Spinal pathology

Investigations

- Wall test – diminished spine extension means that the patient's occiput, scapula, buttocks and heels cannot contact the wall simultaneously.
- Bloods – seronegative for rheumatoid factor.
- Radiology – chest x-ray and MRI to assess changes in the spine.

Treatment

- Conservative: patient education. Refer to physiotherapy.
- Medical: analgesia (NSAIDs) and DMARDs (e.g. sulphasalazine [first line]).
- Surgical: corrective spinal surgery.

Complications

- Osteoporosis.
- Spinal fractures.
- Increased risk of cardiovascular disease (e.g. stroke and myocardial infarction).

Treatment

- Conservative: physiotherapy.
- Medical: effective analgesia.
- Surgical: laminectomy.

Complications

- Paralysis.
- Incontinence.
- Difficulty balancing.

Map 8.7. Hip pathology

MAP 8.7. **Hip pathology**

Proximal femoral fracture

What is a proximal femoral fracture?

Fractures may be defined as a discontinuity of bone and, where the proximal femur is concerned, it usually occurs in the elderly and is more common in women.

The fracture may be defined as extracapsular or intracapsular. Intracapsular fractures are further subdivided into sub-capital and trans-cervical types, whereas extracapsular fractures may be categorized as basi-cervical, inter-trochanteric and sub-trochanteric. There is a high risk of avascular necrosis with intracapsular fractures. The blood supply of the proximal femur is from:

1. The medial femoral circumflex artery.
2. The lateral femoral circumflex artery.
3. The artery of the ligamentum teres.

Causes

- Pathological fracture – osteoporosis, metastases to bone.
- Trauma.

Slipped upper femoral epiphysis

What is slipped upper femoral epiphysis (SUFE)?

This is a rare condition in which the upper femoral epiphysis slips posteroinferiorly from the femoral neck. It may occur bilaterally in 20% of cases. It is very difficult to diagnose.

Causes

- Cartilaginous physis failure.

Risk factors

Include:
- Obesity.
- Male sex.
- Endocrine imbalances (e.g. hypothyroidism, decreased sex hormones).

Symptoms

- Pain – tends to be localized to the knee and thigh.
- Decreased leg abduction, increased adduction, slight leg shortening and external rotation. Loss of internal rotation.

Investigations

- Radiology – x-ray. Severity is assessed using the Southwick angle.

Treatment

- External in-situ pinning or open reduction and pinning.

Complications

- Chondrolysis.
- Deformity.
- Osteoarthritis.
- Avascular necrosis – high risk from reduction of SUFE.

Continued overleaf

Symptoms

- Pain.
- Shortening of the affected leg.
- External rotation of the affected leg.

Investigations

- Routine pre-operative blood tests.
- Radiology – x-ray. The Garden classification is used to describe proximal intracapsular femoral fractures:
  - Type I: undisplaced.
  - Type II: undisplaced but complete fracture.
  - Type III: displaced fracture but still bony contact.
  - Type IV: completely displaced.

Treatment

- Extracapsular fractures:
  - Dynamic hip screw.
- Intracapsular fractures:
  - Undisplaced: internal fixation or hemiarthroplasty.
  - Displaced: hemiarthroplasty or total hip replacement.

Complications

- Avascular necrosis.
- Thromboembolism.
- Complications associated with fractures (see Tables 8.1a, b, pp. 220, 221).

Map 8.7 Hip pathology

Map 8.7. Hip pathology

MAP 8.7. **Hip pathology** (*continued*)

Perthes disease

What is Perthes disease?

This is also known as Legg-Calvé-Perthes disease and is osteonecrosis of the femoral head resulting in deformation of the epiphysis (fragmentation and flattening). There are three phases in the disease process:

1. Initial – crescent shaped femoral head.
2. Resorption – rarefaction (Gage's sign on x-ray – a V shaped lucency).
3. Reparative.

Causes
Unknown

Symptoms
- Child with a limp (boys affected more than girls).
- Hip pain, which may radiate to the knee and groin.
- Decreased range of hip movement.

Developmental dysplasia of the hip

What is developmental dysplasia of the hip (DDH)?

This ranges from mild dysplasia to irreducible dislocation due to a developmental deformation of the hip joint. Females are affected more than males. The condition may be bilateral.

Causes

The exact cause of this condition is unknown but several risk factors have been identified such as:

- Female sex.
- First born child.
- Breech delivery.
- Oligohydramnios.
- Positive family history.
- Ethnicity: Caucasian and North American Indians.

DDH is associated with:

- Congenital talipes equinovarus.
- Torticollis.
- Metatarsus adductus.

Symptoms

- Asymptomatic.
- Asymmetric gluteal skin folds.
- Limp.

Investigations

- DDH screening.
- Ortolani's and Barlow's test.
- Radiology – USS.

Treatment

Depends on age of diagnosis

- Closed reduction: Pavlik harness, hip spica.
- Open reduction: derotation varus osteotomy, Salter osteotomy.

Complications

- Gait abnormalities.
- Limb shortening.
- External rotation of the foot.

Investigations

- Radiology – x-ray. May show several features (e.g. **ABC**):
  - **A** – Abnormal physeal growth
  - **B** – Bone density increased at epiphysis
  - **C** – Calcification lateral to epiphysis

Treatment

- Conservative: physiotherapy, brace, traction.
- Medical: adequate analgesia.
- Surgical: femoral +/- pelvic osteotomy.

Complications

- Gait abnormalities.
- Arthritis.

Map 8.7. Hip pathology

TABLE 8.2. **Knee pathology. The knee is susceptible to both primary and secondary osteoarthritis, but the stability of the knee rests upon intra- and extra-articular ligaments and menisci, which are susceptible to injury.**

Pathology	Cause	Symptoms	Investigations	Treatment	Complications
Anterior cruciate ligament (ACL) tear	The function of the ACL is to: 1. Prevent anterior displacement of the tibia off the femur 2. Prevent rotation 3. Prevent hyperextension Any type of trauma that involves twisting of a slightly flexed knee (e.g. football injuries, or over-extension of the knee) can damage the ACL Females (post puberty) are more likely to damage their ACL than males. The reason for this is debated but is potentially due to: • Hormones – which cause laxity of ligaments • A narrower intercondylar notch • A larger Q angle in women	• Pain • Knee swelling • Hearing or feeling a 'pop'	• Anterior draw test positive/Lachman test positive • Pivot shift test • Radiology: ○ x-ray – rule out fracture ○ MRI – confirms diagnosis	**Conservative:** Employ **RICE** techniques (Rest, Ice, Compression and Elevation), physiotherapy, knee brace **Medical:** analgesia **Surgical:** ACL reconstruction	• Knee instability • Osteoarthritis • Complications relating to surgery such as the general complications of anaesthesia, infection, DVT, damage to surrounding structures

Table 8.2. Knee pathology

| Posterior cruciate ligament (PCL) tear | The function of the PCL is to prevent posterior displacement of the tibia off the femur

Injury to the PCL is very rare. It tends to occur in road traffic accident dashboard injuries | • Pain
• Knee swelling | • Positive posterior draw test
• Radiology:
 ○ x-ray – rule out fracture
 ○ MRI – confirms diagnosis | **Conservative:**
Employ **RICE** techniques (Rest, Ice, Compression and Elevation), physiotherapy, knee brace
Medical: analgesia
Surgical: PCL reconstruction | • Knee instability
• Osteoarthritis
• Complications relating to surgery such as the general complications of anaesthesia, infection, DVT, damage to surrounding structures |

Continued overleaf

Table 8.2: Knee pathology

Table 8.2. Knee pathology

TABLE 8.2. Knee pathology. The knee is susceptible to both primary and secondary osteoarthritis, but the stability of the knee rests upon intra- and extra-articular ligaments and menisci, which are susceptible to injury *(continued)*.

Pathology	Cause	Symptoms	Investigations	Treatment	Complications
Meniscal tears	The medial meniscus is torn more often then the lateral meniscus. The reason for this rests in anatomical differences. The medial meniscus is firmly attached to both the medial collateral ligament and joint capsule. It is also more C shaped in contrast with the lateral meniscus, which is round in appearance Trauma as a result of twisting is the common mechanism of injury. Tears may be categorized as complete or incomplete The combination of a medial meniscus tear, medial collateral ligament tear and a torn ACL is known as O'Donoghue's unhappy triad	• Knee locking • Giving way of the knee • Pain • Swelling • Decreased range of movement	• Positive McMurray test • Radiology: ○ x-ray – rule out fracture ○ MRI – confirms diagnosis	**Conservative:** Employ RICE techniques (Rest, Ice, Compression and Elevation), physiotherapy, knee brace **Medical:** analgesia **Surgical:** depends on the location and the extent of the tear. If located in the outer third of the meniscus, also known as the 'red zone', the tear will heal on its own since this is a region of copious blood supply. However, if located in the inner two thirds, the 'white zone', patients may require surgical intervention	• Knee instability • Osteoarthritis

Osgood–Schlatter disease	This is a tibial tuberosity apophysitis that typically affects athletic males aged 10–15 years The exact cause is not known but overuse is thought to play a role	• Pain, swelling and tenderness of the tibial tuberosity	• Usually a clinical diagnosis • Radiology – x-ray may show signs of tuberosity enlargement	**Conservative:** rest, physiotherapy, knee brace **Medical:** analgesia	• Unlikely to cause serious complications but pain may persist

Osteo-chondritis dissecans	This is a partial or complete detachment of either bone or articular cartilage that is caused by avascular necrosis of the subchondral bone.
	This results in microfracture without remodelling
	
	Other causes include:
	• Genetics
	• Repetitive minor trauma
	• Drugs (e.g. steroids)
		• Pain – worsens with exercise
		• Swelling
		• Locking and giving way
			• Radiology:
			  ○ x-ray – rule out fracture
			  ○ MRI – confirms diagnosis
			
			The Anderson staging criteria are employed
				Conservative: watchful waiting, rest
				
				Medical: analgesia
				
				Surgical: arthroscopy, osteochondral autograft transplantation
					• Osteoarthritis

Patellar sub-luxation syndrome	Exact cause is unknown but some factors have been suggested such as: • Gait abnormalities • Shallow patellar groove • Wide pelvis This condition is more common in women	• Knee that gives way or locks during movement • Sliding and highly mobile patella • Pain – when sitting and worsens with movement • Swelling	• Radiology: x-ray, MRI	**Conservative:** physiotherapy, braces, orthotics **Medical:** analgesia **Surgical:** medial patellofemoral ligament reconstruction. This ligament may tear when the patella dislocates outwards	• Knee instability • Recurrent subluxation or dislocation

Table 8.2. Knee pathology

Table 8.3. Foot pathology

TABLE 8.3. **Foot pathology.**

Pathology	Cause	Symptoms	Investigations	Treatment	Complications
Hallux valgus (bunion)	The exact cause is unknown but it is associated with: • Female sex • Positive family history • Increased age • Wearing heels	• The hallux deviates laterally at the metatarsophalangeal joint • Pain • Erythematous, irritated skin overlying the bunion	• Thorough physical examination including an assessment of gait • Radiology: x-ray will visualize the deformity	**Conservative:** appropriate footwear **Medical:** analgesia **Surgical:** only indicated if there is severe pain or if the deformity significantly impacts on walking/lifestyle	• Osteoarthritis • Complications relating to surgery such as infection, DVT, damage to surrounding structures
Pes planus	Collapse of the medial longitudinal arch	• Asymptomatic • Pain – over the tibialis posterior tendon • Progressed disease – inability to raise heel. Forefoot – abducted; hindfoot – valgus	• Paediatrics – foot proforma • Thorough physical examination including an assessment of gait • Radiology: x-ray may help evaluate the extent of the deformity	Most are asymptomatic and do not require treatment **Conservative:** orthotics, physiotherapy (e.g. Achilles tendon stretching) **Surgical:** in severe cases and aims to realign the foot. Example operations include Achilles tendon lengthening, tibialis posterior tendon reconstruction and reconstructive osteotomies	• Tibialis posterior tendon dysfunction • May contribute to other foot conditions such as hallux valgus and plantar fasciitis

Pes cavus	The exact cause of the accentuated longitudinal arch in this condition is unknown, but is associated with conditions such as: • Cerebral palsy • Spina bifida • Muscular dystrophy • Charcot–Marie–Tooth disease	• Pain on walking • Claw toes • Ankle instability	• Paediatrics – foot proforma • Thorough physical examination including an assessment of gait • Radiology: x-ray may help evaluate the extent of the deformity	**Conservative:** orthotics, physiotherapy **Surgical:** plantar fascia release, Jones procedure, extensor shift procedure, Girdlestone-Taylor transfer, peroneus longus to peroneus brevis tenodesis	• Complications relating to surgery such as infection, DVT, damage to surrounding structures, malunion
Stress fracture	Fractures tend to affect the shaft of the 2nd or 3rd metatarsal since these are less robust than the other metatarsal bones	• Pain on walking and over the metatarsal	• Radiology: x-ray	**Conservative:** rest, plaster cast may be required **Medical:** analgesia	• Complications of fracture (see Tables 8.1a, b, pp. 220, 221) • Osteoarthritis
Talipes equino-varus (club foot)	The exact cause of this condition is unknown but it is associated with: • A positive family history • DDH • Oligohydramnios • Spina bifida	• Inverted and supinated foot • Adducted forefoot • Inwardly rotated heel held in plantarflexion	• USS screening during pregnancy • Diagnosis based on typical appearance • Investigate underlying cause	Ponseti method	• Gait abnormaility • Arthritis • Smaller shoe size of affected foot

Table 8.3 Foot pathology

MAP 8.8. Orthopaedic infections

MAP 8.8. **Orthopaedic infections**

Septic arthritis

What is septic arthritis?
This is infection of any joint by a microorganism. It is a surgical emergency.

Causes
The exact mechanism by which the organism invades the joint is unknown. Spread may be systemic, from a penetrating wound or from prior osteomyelitis.

Causative organisms include:
- *Staphylococcus aureus* (commonest).
- *Neisseria gonorrhoea.*
- *Haemophilus influenzae.*
- *Pneumococcus* sp.
- Group B streptococci.
- *Escherichia coli.*
- *Pseudomonas* sp.
- *Proteus* sp.
- Fungi.

Septic arthritis is associated with:
- Diabetes mellitus.
- IV drug abuse.
- Extremes of age (i.e. the very young/old).

Osteomyelitis

What is osteomyelitis?
This is a bacterial infection of the bone, which may be spread to the bone haematogenously, traumatically or from infection of soft tissue. It may have an acute or chronic presentation.

Causes
Causative organisms include:
- *Staphylococcus aureus* (commonest).
- *Haemophilus influenzae* (more common in children).
- *Salmonella* sp. (more common in patients with sickle cell disease).

Osteomyelitis is associated with:
- Diabetes mellitus.
- IV drug abuse.
- Extremes of age (i.e. the very young/old).
- Sickle cell disease.
- Immunocompromise.
- Chronic osteomyelitis – smoking, steroid use and vascular disease.

Symptoms
- General features of infection: pyrexia, malaise.
- Decreased range of movement of affected joint.
- Inflammation and pain of affected joint.

Symptoms

- General features of infection: spiking pyrexia, malaise
- Decreased range of movement of affected joint
- Inflammation and pain of affected joint

Investigations

- Blood tests – FBC, WCC, U&E, CRP, blood cultures, uric acid to exclude gout.
- Specific tests – joint aspiration and culture, gonorrhoea swabs.
- Radiology:
  - x-ray of joint (and chest if TB suspected).
  - USS – allows diagnostic joint aspiration.

Treatment

This must be done without delay since septic arthritis is an emergency.
Surgical: joint aspiration and surgical washout followed by antibiotics sensitive to causative organism.

Complications

- Joint destruction.
- Secondary osteoarthritis.
- Fibrous ankylosis.
- In children – growth disruption from growth plate damage.

Investigations

- Blood tests – FBC, WCC, CRP, ESR, blood cultures, uric acid to exclude gout.
- Specific tests – joint aspiration and culture.
- Radiology:
  - x-ray of joint (no abnormal features in the first 10–14 days).
  - USS – allows diagnostic joint aspiration.
  - CT – may be used to guide needle aspiration.
  - MRI.

Treatment

- Conservative: splintage, rehabilitation and physiotherapy.
- Medical: IV antibiotics.
- Surgical: guided aspiration and surgical evacuation.

Complications

- Joint destruction.
- Chronic osteoarthritis.
- Septic arthritis.
- Pathological fracture.
- In children – growth disruption from growth plate damage.

MAP 8.8. Orthopaedic infections

Figure 8.2. The lumbar plexus

FIGURE 8.2. **The lumbar plexus**

Deep fibular nerve:
Tibialis anterior
Extensor hallicus longus
Fibularis tertius
Extensor digitorum longus and brevis

Superficial fibular nerve:
Fibularis longus and brevis

Lateral plantar nerve:
Those not supplied by medial plantar nerve

Medial plantar nerve:
Abductor hallicus
Flexor digitorum brevis
Flexor hallicus brevis

Femoral nerve:
anterior compartment of thigh

Obturator nerve:
medial compartment of thigh

Perineal nerve:
Perineum

L2
L3
L4
L5
S1
S2
S3
S4

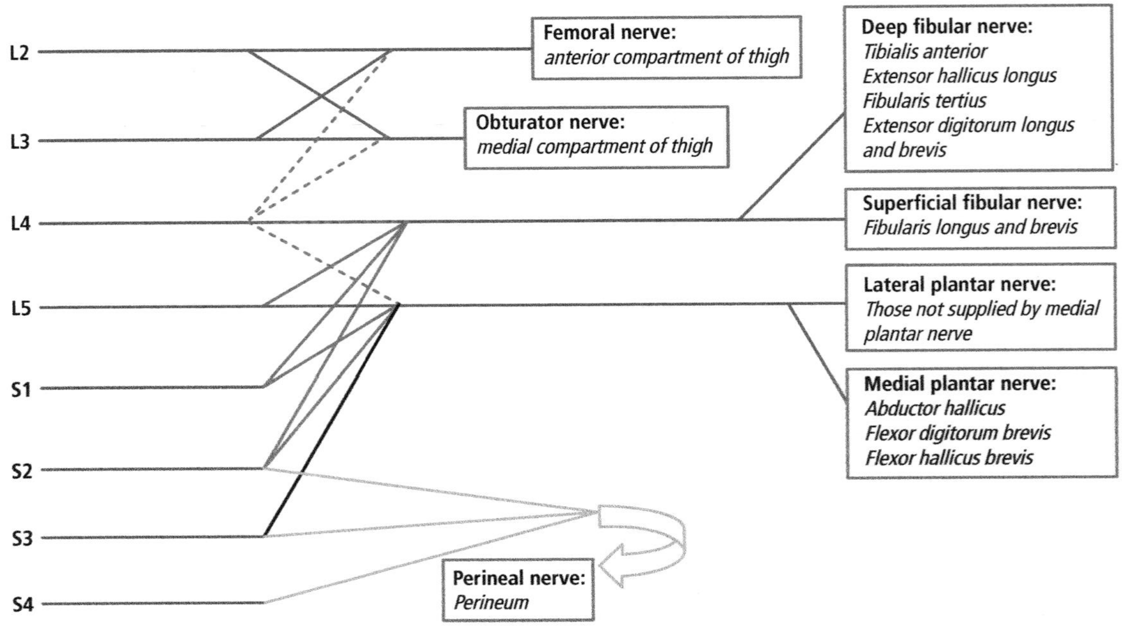

Classification	Name of disease
DSM-5, ICD-10	Psychiatric disorders
HADS, PHQ-9, GAD-7	Depression
SCOFF questionnaire	Anorexia nervosa/bulimia
ACE-III	Dementia
Amsel's criteria	Bacterial vaginosis
Rotherham criteria	Polycystic ovary syndrome
FIGO	Obstetric malignancy staging system
Jones criteria	Rheumatic fever
Duke criteria	Infective endocarditis
Psoriasis Area and Severity Index	Psoriasis
Ludwig scale/Norwood scale	Alopecia
Clark levels and Breslow's thickness	Malignant melanoma
Salter–Harris classification	Growth plate fracture
Garden classification	Proximal femur fracture

DSM-5, Diagnostic and Statistical Manual of Mental Disorders, 5th Edition; ICD-10, International Statistical Classification of Diseases and Related Health Problems, 10th Revision; HADS, Hospital Anxiety and Depression Scale; PHQ-9, Patient Health Questionnaire; GAD-7, Generalized Anxiety Disorder 7; SCOFF, Sick, Control, One stone, Fat, Food; ACE-III, Addenbrooke's Cognitive Examination; FIGO, Fédération Internationale de Gynécologie et d'Obstétrique.

Disease	Website
Acne vulgaris	http://cks.nice.org.uk/acne-vulgaris
Age-related macular degeneration	https://www.rcophth.ac.uk/wp-content/uploads/2014/12/2013-SCI-318-RCOphth-AMD-Guidelines-Sept-2013-FINAL-2.pdf
Alopecia areata	http://cks.nice.org.uk/alopecia-areata
Amenorrhoea	http://cks.nice.org.uk/amenorrhoea
Antepartum haemorrhage	https://www.rcog.org.uk/globalassets/documents/guidelines/gtg63_05122011aph.pdf
Anxiety disorders	https://www.nice.org.uk/guidance/qs53
Bacterial meningitis	http://pathways.nice.org.uk/pathways/bacterial-meningitis-and-meningococcal-septicaemia
Benign paroxysmal positioning disorder	http://cks.nice.org.uk/benign-paroxysmal-positional-vertigo
	http://www.aafp.org/dam/AAFP/documents/patient_care/clinical_recommendations/RecToBOD-020810-Attachment1BPPV-Jan2010Cluster.pdf
Bipolar disorder	https://www.nice.org.uk/guidance/cg38
Borderline personality disorder	https://www.nice.org.uk/guidance/cg78
Bronchiolitis	https://www.nice.org.uk/guidance/ng9
Cataracts	https://www.nice.org.uk/guidance/indevelopment/gid-cgwave0741
	https://www.rcophth.ac.uk/wp-content/uploads/2014/12/2010-SCI-069-Cataract-Surgery-Guidelines-2010-SEPTEMBER-2010.pdf
Cervical cancer	http://cks.nice.org.uk/cervical-cancer-and-hpv
Cervical screening	http://cks.nice.org.uk/cervical-screening
Childhood cancers	http://cks.nice.org.uk/childhood-cancers-recognition-and-referral
Cough in children	http://cks.nice.org.uk/cough-acute-with-chest-signs-in-children
Croup	http://cks.nice.org.uk/croup
Depression	https://www.nice.org.uk/guidance/cg90
Eating disorders	https://www.nice.org.uk/guidance/cg9
Ectopic pregnancy and miscarriage	https://www.nice.org.uk/guidance/cg154
Eczema	http://cks.nice.org.uk/eczema-atopic
Endometrial cancer	http://www.esmo.org/Guidelines/Gynaecological-Cancers/Endometrial-Cancer

Disease	Website
Endometriosis	http://cks.nice.org.uk/endometriosis
Epilepsy	http://cks.nice.org.uk/epilepsy
Epistaxis	http://cks.nice.org.uk/epistaxis-nosebleeds
Gestational trophoblastic disease	https://www.rcog.org.uk/globalassets/documents/guidelines/gt38managementgestational0210.pdf
Glaucoma	https://www.nice.org.uk/guidance/cg85
Hearing loss	https://www.nice.org.uk/guidance/indevelopment/gid-cgwave0833
Hip fracture	https://www.nice.org.uk/guidance/cg124
	https://www.nice.org.uk/guidance/cg124/evidence/full-guideline-183081997
Hot swollen joints/ septic arthritis	http://bestpractice.bmj.com/best-practice/monograph/486/treatment/guidelines.html
Infertility	http://cks.nice.org.uk/infertility
Ménière's disease	http://cks.nice.org.uk/menieres-disease
Menorrhagia	http://cks.nice.org.uk/menorrhagia
Non-complex fractures	https://www.nice.org.uk/guidance/NG38/documents/fractures-full-guideline2
Osteomyelitis	http://bestpractice.bmj.com/best-practice/monograph/354/diagnosis.html
Paediatric diabetes	https://www.nice.org.uk/guidance/ng18
Paediatric urinary tract infection	https://www.nice.org.uk/guidance/cg54
Pityriasis rosea	http://cks.nice.org.uk/pityriasis-rosea
Pityriasis versicolor	http://cks.nice.org.uk/pityriasis-versicolor
Polycystic ovarian syndrome	http://cks.nice.org.uk/polycystic-ovary-syndrome
Postpartum haemorrhage	https://www.rcog.org.uk/globalassets/documents/guidelines/gt52postpartumhaemorrhage0411.pdf
Psoriasis	http://cks.nice.org.uk/psoriasis
Rosacea	http://cks.nice.org.uk/rosacea-acne
Schizophrenia	https://www.nice.org.uk/guidance/cg82
Shoulder dystocia	https://www.rcog.org.uk/globalassets/documents/guidelines/gtg_42.pdf
Vaginal discharge	http://cks.nice.org.uk/vaginal-discharge